Living with Mild Brain Injury

T0373575

This important book presents a unique, personal account of the impact a mild traumatic brain injury can have. It tells the story of Pauline, who was 33 when a late football tackle caused a bleed in her brain which went undiscovered for 18 months. The account includes descriptions of hidden symptoms of concussion and post-concussion syndrome, pitfalls in diagnoses, the uneven progress of recovery and the effect of the varied reactions which others have to an acquired brain injury.

The author incorporates memories alongside extracts from clinic notes, diary entries and emails to reflect the disjointed progress of diagnosis and recovery as – although similar – no two head injuries are the same. Through this book, the reader gains an appreciation of the confusion experienced by many brain injury survivors, which sheds light on why some may develop unusual behaviour or mental health issues, and how such issues can be alleviated. Brain injuries are poorly understood by the general public and this can lead to difficult interactions. Moreover, complications in diagnosis means some may not realise they have this milder form of brain injury.

This book will enlighten brain injury survivors and affected families and allow professionals an insight into their patients' experiences. As concerns grow over the risks which contact sports pose, this book shows how even mild brain injuries can wreak havoc with careers, relationships and one's sense of self, but that a happy life can still be found.

Pauline O'Connor grew up in New Zealand where she gained a degree in Viticulture and Winemaking. She emigrated to London where a football (soccer) tackle led to a bleed in her brain. Pauline began writing during her recovery and documents her experience here and on the website: www.pigpen.page

After Brain Injury: Survivor Stories

This new series of books is aimed at those who have suffered a brain injury, and their families and carers. Each book focuses on a different condition, such as face blindness, amnesia and neglect, or diagnosis, such as encephalitis and locked-in syndrome, resulting from brain injury. Readers will learn about life before the brain injury, the early days of diagnosis, the effects of the brain injury, the process of rehabilitation, and life now. Alongside this personal perspective, professional commentary is also provided by a specialist in neuropsychological rehabilitation, making the books relevant for professionals working in rehabilitation such as psychologists, speech and language therapists, occupational therapists, social workers and rehabilitation doctors. They will also appeal to clinical psychology trainees and undergraduate and graduate students in neuropsychology, rehabilitation science, and related courses who value the case study approach.

With this series, we also hope to help expand awareness of brain injury and its consequences. The World Health Organisation has recently acknowledged the need to raise the profile of mental health issues (with the WHO Mental Health Action Plan 2013–20) and we believe there needs to be a similar focus on psychological, neurological and behavioural issues caused by brain disorder, and a deeper understanding of the importance of rehabilitation support. Giving a voice to these survivors of brain injury is a step in the right direction.

Series Editor: Barbara A. Wilson

Published titles:

Life and Suicide Following Brain Injury
A Personal and Professional Account
Alyson Norman

Adjusting to Brain Injury
Reflections from Survivors, Family Members and Clinicians
Katherine Dawson with Karl Hargreaves, Ashraf Sheikh, Lisa Summerill and Meg Archer

Living with Mild Brain Injury
The Difficulties of Diagnosis and Recovery from Post-Concussion Syndrome
Pauline O'Connor

For more information about this series, please visit: https://www.routledge.com/After-Brain-Injury-Survivor-Stories/book-series/ABI

Living with Mild Brain Injury

The Difficulties of Diagnosis and Recovery from Post-Concussion Syndrome

Pauline O'Connor

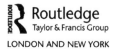

Routledge
Taylor & Francis Group

LONDON AND NEW YORK

First published 2021
by Routledge
2 Park Square, Milton Park, Abingdon, Oxon OX14 4RN

and by Routledge
52 Vanderbilt Avenue, New York, NY 10017

Routledge is an imprint of the Taylor & Francis Group, an informa business

© 2021 Pauline O'Connor

British Library Cataloguing-in-Publication Data
A catalogue record for this book is available from the British Library

Library of Congress Cataloging-in-Publication Data
A catalog record has been requested for this book

ISBN: 978-0-367-52411-1 (hbk)
ISBN: 978-0-367-52408-1 (pbk)
ISBN: 978-1-003-05777-2 (ebk)

Typeset in Times
by SPi Global, India

For 'Ash';

and family & friends,

old & new,

who got me through.

Epigraph

'The message of this lecture is that black holes ain't as black as they are painted. They are not the eternal prisons they were once thought. Things can get out of a black hole, both to the outside, and possibly to another universe. So if you feel you are in a black hole, don't give up. There's a way out.'

Professor Stephen Hawking

Contents

Acknowledgements

A brain injury doesn't happen to a single person. All those around the patient are affected and can influence the recovery in turn. Some people are relied on every hour of the day, some have cameos, while others fade away. Family or friend, acquaintance or stranger, all will shape a brain injury survivor in ways they may never know.

My recovery would have been immeasurably more difficult without the support of family and friends. They have been anonymised throughout this book, and in some cases several friends are merged into a single character. Similarly, I can no longer name the many NHS staff who laid out the diagnostic pathway and cajoled me along it, but I remember your faces well. Along with 'Willow', you get up every day and help others.

Thank you. Thank you to each and every one of you for getting me back to myself.

I am particularly grateful to my writing teacher 'Hawthorn' and to branches of 'Maple' and 'Peony'. Their encouragement and hours of careful editing made this a far better book than I could have managed alone. Without them, I would not have received the memorable feedback: 'This bit is lovely, but where's the rest of the sentence?'

After a busy working day, Dr Barry Seemungal visited his local brain injury charity where he offered knowledge and hope. Then, in the midst of a pandemic, Dr Seemungal and Dr Neil Parrett gave their time and encouragement to a new writer. I am grateful to both for their kindness and expertise.

Finally, my thanks to the BBC, the Stephen Hawking Foundation, United Agents LLP, the New Zealand Herald, NZME, and Headway – the brain injury association – for allowing me to cite their copyrighted material gratis for this project.

Abbreviations

A&E   accident and emergency clinic
ABI   acquired brain injury
CBT   cognitive behavioural therapy
CEO   chief executive officer, the boss of the company
Dr   doctor
FC   football club
GP   General Practitioner
HR   Human Resources
IAM   internal auditory meatus
Kg   kilogram
MRI   magnetic resonance imaging
Neuro   neurological
NHS   National Health Service
PTA   post-traumatic amnesia
St   stone
TBI   traumatic brain injury
Wi-Fi   a wireless connection to the internet.
WTF   what the f*ck

Prologue

22nd of July 2015: Sixteen months after the incident

Bright sunshine hit the water glass and split into a prism of colours which lanced across the cafe. Specks of dust shone in the light, dancing in gentle air currents. I was entranced by the brilliance of a secret ballet suddenly revealed. When a summer cloud moved across the sun, the rainbow of light snapped out. Across the table, Rowan sipped her coffee and I realised that I'd been absent yet again.

I tried to ignore the familiar flush of confused shame and sought to recall what we had been speaking about. These odd moments when my brain would tune out and enter its own gentle world for a while were still happening quite often.

Something would catch my attention and any thought of the present disappeared entirely. It was as if my brain was no longer capable of holding two thoughts at once. Sure, I meant to ask Rowan about her time away. But when the sunbeam turned up, all thoughts of Asia, or indeed of Rowan herself, were just gone.

Rowan, Asia... that's right! Rowan was just back from her secondment and I was struggling to relate to a year that had proved to be so different from my own. And, if I'm completely honest, I was downright jealous of her experience.

'Jealous?' Rowan looked confused.

Great, Now I'm talking out loud too. My shame burned a tad brighter before I could think: *wait, saying that just might help.*

'That's ok,' she reassured me. 'You explained at the start that you might need a quiet moment or two during our conversation. My friend also needs the same thing after his injury.'

Relief flooded in. 'I'm getting better at holding conversations but I still tend to bounce around from topic to topic. I find it hard to keep focus.'

Rowan nodded. 'You know what you are? You are a series of disconnected narratives.'

Usually at this point the writer explains what the injury was, how it happened and just what this recovery is. But that can be a little difficult with brain injuries. Events tend to bleed into each other, just as blood seeps into delicate brain tissue. Large tracts of time are lost, like rain on a window pane eventually soaking up all the individual drops into one long trickle.

Due to the nature of my impaired memory, this story is told through a mixture of medical notes, memories, diary entries, emails and social media posts. The disjointed progress of my diagnosis and treatment meant we never quite knew what was going on. This jumbled path will be familiar to others with brain injury and is reflected in these pages.

I am, however, fortunate to retain a decent memory of the incident. As time has passed it has become easier, and more amusing, to call it that rather than stumble through 'the day a football tackle gave me a traumatic brain injury'.

Sunday, March the 9th 2014. The day of the incident. Although it was not the day my world changed, that came two days later.

2014: Perspective

Chapter 1

Brain injury
The incident and immediate aftermath

Life had followed a fairly standard course: schooling, career, marry high school sweetheart, leave home to travel the world and seek my fortune. There are always variations on this theme, and changes to the best-laid plans.

Much of my schooling involved sports, as many childhoods do in New Zealand. My football career started at eleven years old, when I was granted permission to play in my brother's team. We lived in a small, rural town, and I was the only girl in the league, so they had to create new rules to accommodate me. Right from those early days I cherished the feeling of being a part of a team, of shared endeavour towards a common goal.

Over the next two decades or so, I would play in a dozen different teams, in New Zealand and London. A highlight was playing in the reserve team for a well-known premier league club. No, women weren't paid. In a year in which the club advertised £30million deals for male players, females had to pay a monthly stipend for the right to wear that same jersey.

My initial plans to study geology at university were swayed by a single pamphlet advertising a new course 'Bachelor of Viticulture and Oenology.' What 17-year-old would choose rocks over grape growing and winemaking? I mean, think of the free booze!

The resulting career proved varied. While I did grow grapes and make wine, I also sold, advised and wrote about wine. It can take time to train up the sense of taste and smell to competition level, but over many years of applied effort, I found myself in a role which combined teaching people about wine and helping with international judging events.

In everyone's life, they reach a point when it is either time to settle down where you grew up or travel. My husband, Ash, and I chose the United Kingdom as the first place to visit on our round the world trip. The tour ended quickly when we found ourselves with friends, jobs and enjoying a city lifestyle.

Emigrating half way round the world means you need to meet new people and my first step was to join a local football team, City United. At the first training session I met many new friends. Some bonds were destined to wither while others grew. Hopefully some of those friendships will last for a life time. But you never can tell at first, and few friends are willing to travel the road of trauma and injury with you.

So there I was, in London, playing football, working with wine, still looking for that fortune.

Clinic notes: Pre-incident

Employment: Patient worked full time in a management role which included national and international travel.
Exercise: Cycling 40 miles per week plus weekly football training and matches.
Social: Engagements usually twice a week.
Prior incidents:

- Two diagnosed concussions, one each in 1998 and 2001.
- Both concussions also resulted from impact to the face and nose.
- Patient experienced no complications beyond 24 hours on either occasion.

Sunday the 9th of March: The day of the incident

It was a cracking Sunday afternoon, a perfect day for football. City United faced tough opposition. As a centre-back I was frequently under pressure. It was odd that my injury came when there was no pressure at all. I'd already headed the ball clear when the opposition striker leapt at me in a recklessly late tackle. The full force of her airborne body was behind her shoulder as it slammed into the bridge of my nose.

I remember dropping to the ground, my hands clutching at a nose which already felt three sizes too big. My inner commentary kicked in: *OK, that was a bad one.* Even so, I couldn't quite believe the amount of blood which poured through my hands into an expansive puddle on the ground. I have a strong memory of admiring the way the rich red contrasted beautifully with the vivid spring grass.

There was so much blood that my teammates had to wash it into the pitch while I was led, shakily, away. But at the time there was no dizziness, confusion nor unconsciousness.

Monday: Eighteen hours after the incident

'What the hell?'

Exactly what everyone wants their boss to say first thing in the morning. So I grinned back at Alder and added the obligatory, 'Yeah, you should see the other guy.'

My nose felt gigantic and ached despite the ibuprofen taken liberally at breakfast. The swelling had increased overnight. Bright blue and purple bruises surrounded my eyes and nose in a pantomime villain mask. There was only one way to conceal pain and injury this obvious: with laughter.

As the tale underwent numerous retellings over coffee, the striker became larger and my thwarting of her ambitions ever more courageous. The pain increased so the laughter needed to as well. By lunch time, all jokes regarding the resemblance to a panda had been fully explored.

Football mates were also checking in to see how things were going so I obliged:

'My nose is HUGE!! Check out the photo :-)'

'Woof. Hope the other person came off worse!'

'You look cool! Hope u feel ok.'

'Dear god, no offence that looks horrible.'

That last reply must have hit home as my mask slipped a little before humour sprang back:

'None taken, it is horrible! Ach, well. I've given up on concealer at this point.'

That evening was a regular dinner date with friends. We did what people do: enjoy good food, great wine and excellent company. Do I regret the wine given what came next? I used to; especially given I don't remember much of the meal at all. But eventually… well, we can only hold on to so much guilt and still get out of bed in the morning.

Tuesday, the day my world changed: Thirty-six hours after the incident

Pain, nausea, dizziness, confusion. *WTF? Why is the bed spinning? What the hell is happening?* I had flashes of lucid moments which prompted action in fits and starts. Ash left me in bed with a suspected hangover. While he left for work, I moaned something about feeling awful and dropped back to sleep.

An hour or so later the screen of my phone swerved alarmingly under my gaze. I managed to text the office with an apology for my absence before falling back into a horrible dizzy interlude. Sometime later, consciousness re-emerged to say, '*this isn't right, something is horribly wrong*' before again waving a white flag and succumbing to nausea.

Eventually I managed to check my symptoms on the NHS website. The screen flashed an alarming red: Call an ambulance, seek emergency help.

Tsh phsaw, and yet... Anxiety spurred me into action. I couldn't think straight. Something was wrong, the internet says to get help urgently. But I didn't want to cause a fuss. So I caught a bus.

Part of me was relieved by the weary receptionist's automatic 'and what seems to be the problem?' People are grumpy and put out by others calling for their attention; all is well with the world.

Another part of me wanted to scream: *I can barely stand. I need to grasp the furniture and walls to stay upright. My face is black and blue below eyes swollen with blood. In what world is this a normal Tuesday morning?*

I guess I must have explained the collision on Sunday and my symptoms to her. I don't really remember. I recall flashes of the visit, slumped gratefully into a plastic chair while minutes slipped away, unfelt and untracked in this new nauseous reality.

There was an x-ray and a harried nurse who explained that there was no obvious break in my nose. But there might be microscopic fractures that couldn't be picked up. Beyond that I just had concussion which needed rest.

'So, what do I do about work?'

'I can't sign you off.'

I waited, expecting more. She typed away on her screen for a while before turning back to me with an impatient 'what?'

'Just rest, any other advice?'

'Rest and plenty of fluids.' It was as though I'd come to A&E with a simple cold and was wasting her time.

'Ok, any idea of how long this will last?'

'I can't sign you off work,' came the robotic response.

'I understand that, I'm just hoping for an idea of how long I'll be feeling like this'.

'I can't sign you off work.'

I clenched my fists against my rising frustration and the whirling in my head. 'Yes, you've said that. How about... leaving the work question, can you let me know how long until I can try football again?'

'Take a week off and some ibuprofen.'

This was the advice given to a woman reporting to A&E with facial injuries and brain injury symptoms severe enough that NHS Direct had recommended an ambulance. I was sent home with a prescription for over-the-counter painkillers.

Clinic notes: A&E

> Patient discharged with:
>
> 1. **Certificate of attendance at Emergency department:**
>   THIS IS NOT A MEDICAL CERTIFICATE.
> 2. **Prescription:** Ibuprofen and paracetamol

Somehow, I captured all this in an email to the City United football coach later that day.

ME: Dizziness all morning → A&E → Concussion and possible hairline fracture(s). Out till at least next Tuesday, possibly longer. Son of a b*tch.

12th to 19th of March: Three to ten days after the incident

The next week was spent at home or in aborted attempts to return to work. I was desperate for the dizzying fog to lift and exhausted from lack of sleep. Sleep was what I really wanted, to disappear into blissful rest and leave this pain behind. Sleep would have been the best thing for my brain too, not for nothing do people refer to the healing powers of sleep.

Sadly, sleep was the one thing I couldn't have. My brain was struggling with the ceaseless whirling. We aren't meant to be dizzy constantly, so my 'fight or flight' response was always engaged. But there was no respite. There was nothing to fight and no way to escape the spinning inside my head.

Instead, I would lie in bed counting the cracks on the ceiling and watching the leaves bud on the tree outside my window. Threadbare branches bending to chilly winds were a desolate companion for the needy.

At one point, while searching for answers, or possibly for something to fight, I looked at the website of the club we had been playing when I was injured. While there were no answers there, I did get an 'ah-ha' moment.

'Anonymous FC is a community club located between two of London's largest and most notorious housing estates.'

Yes, that is really how their own website advertised the team. Another day, I was looking for a new focus for my 'blame ray'. Searing pain and red-hot frustration had combined with flammable anxiety for days, refining them into a tight beam of blame. The ray had flitted from me, to healthcare workers, to alcohol and back to me so often that it needed a new target. I decided to investigate the original tackle further.

Summary of emails with City United coach

ME: Afraid this injury has turned out to be more serious than it appeared. I can't read for a decent length of time without being floored by dizziness. Still very much house bound and haven't managed to get back to work yet. I've not had anything like it before so no idea when I'll be back, I'm afraid. Not sure how much I remember about the 'tackle', but don't think I was knocked out. Did you see much?

CITY UNITED COACH: Wow, I didn't realise it was so bad. I don't really remember much other than what I mentioned at the time. It looked as though the striker jumped into you side on, and then caught you with her shoulder. It was pretty late, so I was already looking at where the ball was going by the time she made contact. Since you didn't lose consciousness or seem dizzy in any way, I didn't think that the impact would be hard enough to cause anything like these sorts of problems. I always thought that a concussion was a doctor's way of saying there are no serious problems, but take it easy for a few days.

ME: Yeah, that was my view on concussion but turns out it means 'injury to the brain that we can't do anything about'.

Hospital redux: Eleven days after the incident

After ten days in bed or on the sofa, I made it back to the office. *Surely if life gets back to normal my head will become normal too – hurray!* Alder, my manager, promptly sent me home.

'You're a zombie' he pronounced and insisted on walking me to the station.

After that, I managed to see my GP for the first of many visits, for the first of many sick notes. She also referred me to another hospital where I presented myself that afternoon. The staff rushed me through to meet their treatment deadlines.

'You should have been here last week.'

'Believe me, had I known this was an option I would have been.'

After a quick check of the nose: 'Yep, that's broken.'
'Oh, the other hospital's A&E told me it wasn't.'
'Really?! You should have had an x-ray.'
'I did.'
'Oh.' There was a silence then, 'Well… at least it's fairly straight. You shouldn't have much of a nasal deformity.'

Nasal deformity – awesome. It speaks to how naive I was at that stage that having a misshapen nose was my main concern. Though in fairness, my career relied on my sense of smell. That it was a source of anxiety was sensible, I just didn't realise there were bigger things to worry about.

There was another wait before a neurological examination which tested my reflexes and responses. I could recite my symptoms quite clearly by now:

* always dizzy even when lying down
* nausea but no vomiting
* constant splitting headache
* fuzzy, foggy brain
* huge trouble with memory and concentration
* walking into things and trouble staying upright but I haven't fallen

I would only work out later that all these symptoms are subjective. If you don't actually vomit or fall over then no one else can see the problem. There is no way for anyone, health worker or otherwise, to see the pain pulsing behind the eyes, to know the fogginess that affects every thought or to understand the effort required to simply walk down an empty corridor.

Clinic notes: Urgent referral

The above-named patient received treatment in the Urgent Referral Clinic today for: Concussion
Treatment Given includes: Neurological examination normal. Reassured – advised to seek medical attention if any concerns
Investigations done: Nil
Plan: Discharge

The note to seek medical attention if any concerns seems absurd. *That's why I was here!* But I cradled the paper with a written diagnosis reverently. My husband greeted me with relief, at last we had an answer. We didn't think it could be wrong.

Chapter 2

Clinical advice and symptoms

Just wait it out

April to... How long will these symptoms last?

Email to Peony: One month after the incident

ME: You have no idea how good it is to hear from you. Orders are to 'do nothing stimulating' and I last left the house a week ago for an exhilarating outing to the hospital. So, things have been boring and lonely during the days, our resident spider is not a conversationalist. Trying to make it back to the office next week so hope to see you soon after that.

It had been a horrible few weeks, but we did have a few answers. Though it wasn't written on the clinic notes, I had been told I had post-concussion syndrome which normally lasts six weeks. I was already in the third week and we tried to find solace in the fact that I was half way there.

I had also received valuable instructions to help the recovery. The specialists said I must rest for a few weeks. My brain needed to stop now to prevent further damage and let the damaged tissue heal. This is a problem, as you need your brain for everything. Essentially, I had to stay in bed and do nothing. No reading, no watching shows or movies, no listening to music. Nothing. For three weeks.

My boss, Alder, took it in his stride. 'Ok, we'll sort the team and your workload out. Take the time you need to heal and we'll speak again in three weeks.'

Relieved, I retreated to bed and to the view of my now favourite tree. Verdant green leaves waved at me in a warm breeze, squirrels leapt about. It seemed so peaceful. I wanted peace, I ached to relax. But how do you rest when everything inside you is crying out? *What the hell is happening to me?!*

I've told you what is happening. I'd told the doctors and nurses at every examination. But some symptoms can hide others, to the extent that even the person experiencing them doesn't notice. This was certainly the case for me, my dizziness hid the extent of my fatigue. It didn't help that the fatigue was all encompassing, I didn't notice the extent of it because the pathological fatigue was always there. We can't tell others of something which we haven't noticed ourselves. And the nature of these symptoms mean they can be difficult even for someone else, even a health professional, to detect.

The main symptoms of brain injury are well documented:

- Dizziness
- Balance issues
- Nausea
- Tinnitus
- Fatigue
- Memory problems
- Headache

But what do they really feel like?

Physical injuries

My most obvious injuries were actually the least worrying. The initial impact had given me impressive bruising and a broken nose. Six weeks after the injury, because of niggling pains in my face, I booked an appointment with my dentist. He found cracked molars and minor fractures in my cheek bones. There wasn't much to be done about the cheek bones but a few fillings were replaced. The black eyes faded over time and the nose healed straight. By the end of the first month, I looked deceptively normal.

Dizziness

Dizziness was my main complaint at the time, mostly because it was constant. Whether I was walking, standing still or laying down I had a sensation of falling sideways for a second before catching myself, then falling again. When my eyes were open this translated to my vision too. Whatever I was looking at would slide diagonally down to the left before springing back into place and sliding again. I have a distant memory of looking at a tiled wall. The tiles would slide down sideways, as if melting off the wall. Then suddenly they were back in their normal place. A second later they began sliding again. Serious concentration was required to bring anything into focus. This was true whether I was looking at a wall, a screen, a person, or if I was trying to cross a busy street.

To give an example, I once became trapped in a bathroom. All I needed to do was turn the lock and I'd be free. But, to my eyes, the door was sliding to the left before springing back to centre and sliding sideways again. The lock seemed to be circling in space and 'catching' it was difficult. In the end, I had to sit on the floor and work my hands up to the handle order to find the lock, and freedom. This movement in my vision meant that reading, writing or typing were nearly impossible. In one email from that time, I noted that just writing 100 words to a friend had taken me a day.

There was no respite. Even when I lay down with my eyes closed the world still spun. Many of my days were spent lying still, but tense. I needed to grip the bed against the constant feeling that it was spinning. My arms and hands ached from clutching the sheets until they would eventually turn numb. In trying to rest I ended up with repetitive strain injuries in my arms and hands.

All of this damage and fear was caused by my brain. It told me we were constantly lurching to the left then spinning back in a macabre ballet of sensations. There was nothing I could do but lie rigid, trying to avoid sinking into the ever-present primal fear that this was all I could ever manage to do again. After hours of counting the whirling circuits in my head I would, on a good day, sink into the welcoming black hole of exhausted sleep.

Nausea

I felt sick, on the edge of vomiting, most of the time. Was it from the dizziness and associated vertigo? I didn't know and it seemed there wasn't much I could do about this one. I had been given a prescription for anti-nausea pills after my second visit to A&E and took it to the hospital pharmacist.

'Could you confirm you address please?'

Once I had done so, she continued:

'I need to tell you about some of the side effects of this drug. The common ones people might get are headaches, dizziness…'

I regret that I cut her off with a curse. 'Sorry, but I already have plenty of those.'

She looked at the letter. 'Post-concussion syndrome. Ah. Well, this is only prescribed to help you with the nausea so if you'd rather not take them?'

'Can I just get more of the painkillers please?'

At the time, this was one of the more manageable symptoms. I ate when my stomach allowed. Oddly, despite the nausea, I was starving. My brain was struggling to heal and to continue to function at the same time. It was as though I was 'eating for two', one meal for me, another for my brain. It wasn't just food; I drank far more water than I usually did. Somehow, this food and water actually helped the nausea, I often felt ill before a meal but seldom afterwards.

Balance issues

During one of my depressingly regular visits to my GP for a sick note, we also discussed my balance problems. In the weeks after the incident, I was walking into things, struggling to stand steady when tired, and collapsing when trying to get up from sitting or lying. More frequent were the times when I would catch myself, only just managing to stay upright.

When I was up and about, I'd forget about my limbs and would often walk into the door jam or the low coffee table. My shoulders, elbows and knees were spotted with bruises at various stages of healing. Or I'd reach for something with one hand and the other would knock over an aisle display because it wanted to play along too. It felt like the map in my head of how big my body was and where everything was had large empty spaces: 'here be dragons'.

On the GP's recommendation I started tai chi that week. I wasn't expecting much, but then that is usually when one is most surprised. After my first lesson I bumped into fewer things. As the lessons continued, my bruises faded and I was able to stand steadier each day. The lessons were tiring though. I'd need a nap just to get the energy to go to bed.

Tweet
Second tai chi class, and a noticeable improvement in balance and co-ordination – woo hoo. Starting to hope that the brain is on the mend :)

Tinnitus

Every now and then before the incident, I would notice a faint buzz in my ear. Just a little whirr when things were really quiet. I'd looked it up and found that about a third of people experience tinnitus at some point in their lives. It would go away again and I wouldn't worry about it.

Tinnitus came back with a vengeance as part of my brain injury symptoms. This time it was an invasive high-pitched whine, like I was being tracked by a drone. Another thing to keep me awake. Another thing to grit the teeth against and try to ignore. Just when I'd managed to reduce the persistent hum to a background noise the damned thing would change tone! It was infuriating. In the very moment I found a little space my nemesis shifted to another form. It was enough to drive me to tears, and it often did.

I spent long hours looking out of my bedroom window because a high-pitched whine was keeping me from doing anything else. Pillows were soaked with tears as I would choose whether to focus on the whirling dizziness behind my eyelids or the buzzing in my head. At night, Ash would wake to find me clutching my head, crying in angry exhaustion and would do his best to calm us both to sleep. Sleep, or rather its absence, became my prime concern. It was more important than food, or my husband or even me. *Sleep, where the f*ck have you gone?*

Fatigue

To paraphrase, no two brain injuries are the same, but they do rhyme. A constant rhythm in the lives of most brain injury survivors is the need to deal with fatigue. And we aren't talking just being tired. The pathological fatigue after a brain injury is nothing like that felt after a long shift or a big weekend. It is not a weariness which can be resolved with one or two good nights of sleep.

Pathological fatigue is a constant companion. Sleep might alleviate it to some extent but it is never dismissed. This fatigue sits like a dust sheet over the body, muffling sensations and slowing movements. It is easy to describe the physical effects.

'Walking is like wading through concrete' or 'limbs feel heavy as lead.'

The real effect of fatigue is in the brain. Thoughts which used to zip around without a problem are stuck on an interminable Sunday bus service. Picking up a cup, something I had managed to do without thought for over thirty years, now required the concentration and attention of a chess grandmaster. Imagine if every time you wanted a sip of tea you had to concentrate on every single movement:

1. Locate the cup. Sounds easy but don't forget your dizziness interferes with your vision so it takes a few seconds to come into focus.
2. Move your arm and towards the cup. Careful now, the tea is hot and your arm is heavy. So heavy. It feels like if you drop your arm it would break the wooden table.

3. Ok, got there. Now get your index finger through the handle, and grip. You used to have strength once.
4. Right, deep breath, and lift your arm up. Whoops, need to keep the cup steady. No spilling, that would mean more effort to tidy it up. Good, you got there.
5. Time to tilt the cup gently, your arm is aching but you can do this. Co-ordinate though, tilt it when your lips are open but you aren't inhaling. Don't want to choke again.

The effort of concentration means you are sweating, but you can't col- lapse yet. You have to do the whole thing in reverse before you can rest. You need to do all that just to sip some tea. Imagine cooking a whole meal.

One month after the incident I was averaging eighteen hours sleep a day and something as simple as taking a shower would wear me out. Even dur- ing my six waking hours, naps were frequent and all I could manage were basic survival tasks. *Food, water, shower, bed. No, I can't manage the shower too, I'll have to have a nap first.*

But here is the kicker, I didn't realise how tired I was.

This fatigue was always there so I simply didn't see it. For a year. Time and again Ash would have to tell me to go to bed. I was so fatigued that even recognising the fatigue was beyond me. It was only when I looked back from a year on, that I realised just how bloody hard it had been.

Many of the other problems I encountered over the first year of my recovery were linked directly to this fatigue. As I learned how to manage it, my other symptoms improved dramatically.

Memory and brain fog

Problems with knowledge retention and memory are probably one of the most obvious, and frustrating, symptoms when you are caring for some- one with a brain injury. Trust me, they can be just as frustrating for the person with the injury too, only with an added frisson of fear. *Sh*t, he did tell me that. Why didn't I remember? What's wrong with me? Why can't I do simple things any more. Will I ever be able to remember anything ever again? Wait, he's been speaking again. What did he say?*

It isn't that I'm deliberately ignoring you or forgetting all these impor- tant things. It's just that my brain is busy. It is fighting the dizziness to try to keep me upright. It is struggling to remember where the counter top is so that I don't drop the mug on the floor. It is trying not to worry about having to consciously do all that in order to just survive. It is summoning up the energy from somewhere to do all these things.

I need to tell you that I'm sorry I missed what you said and I didn't mean for you to have to repeat yourself for a third time. But I just don't have brain space or the energy to remember to do that either. And now you've gone. *I wanted to say something, but so tired. He's annoyed, I know. But I can't remember why. He wanted me to do something. I need to do something. The kitchen is spinning again...*

In the fatigued fog of these early months, I have a clear memory from a single morning. It is odd the things that stick in the mind. I was struggling to get to an appointment but the walk to the bus stop was proving an epic challenge. *It's only 40 metres away now.* I kept my eyes fixed on it while I forced one dizzy step after the other, closer and closer. *Not so far now after all the way I've walked.* A bus whooshed passed and shuddered to a halt in front of the sign. *Only 30 metres now, I can definitely make it.* There is a lady with a pram getting off and a man stooped over his cane working up the effort to step up through the door. He's taking his time, time I'll need to get there. *20 metres, I can't miss this bus I'll be late.*

As the bus pulled away from the stop, I realised the game was up. I couldn't even manage a quick step ten metres to catch a bus; there was no way my plans for the day were going to happen. I wasn't ready for the world yet. My house, my sofa and my bed were the only safe places.

Summary of emails with Laurel

ME: Getting back into the world is still very slow, I couldn't even catch a bus today. All the advice from GP and specialist advice services have been 'yes, it is slow but there is nothing else we can do'. Seems very odd but I am improving and they keep saying I don't need a scan or other treatment.

LAUREL: Have you emailed that lady about Reiki yet? I know it's hippy-like, but every little helps and all that.

Now I may be in need of help and desperate for something, anything, to get me out of this horrible nightmare brain-scape of dizziness and fatigue. But I'm a doctor's daughter with a firm belief in science and medicine. I wasn't about to head off for some weird laying on of hands where someone transfers energy in to me. I had enough nervous energy of my own to deal with right now.

And yet I was doing tai chi. Religiously. My weekly lessons and daily practise were a priority because they helped. Ash thought that the movements helped as they gave me something to focus on. I suspected that the slow repetitive movements were helping my addled brain to re-build the spatial map of my body and its presence in space. Whatever it was, it worked. I was calmer and walking was easier.

So while I dismissed Reiki, I still wondered *am I missing something else that might help? Let's face it, I really need help.* Which is why, after months of struggling to get my life back together, I joined Peony at an introductory meditation class. If nothing else, it was a break from the four walls I was stuck between most days now.

That was how I found myself propped up on cushions on a polished floor listening to the drone in my head fight with the noise of busy traffic outside. I was supposed to be concentrating on my breathing but the brain couldn't settle. *How can I possibly sit still thinking about nothing but breathing for an hour?* I'd been in Britain long enough to prefer to endure rather than make a scene by walking out. Resigned to staying still, and sure that eventually my feet would just go numb, I carried on.

The minutes of silence ticked by and slowly my thoughts stopped racing. The fear and anxiety dropped from fever pitch. In the brief calm I realised that there, hidden behind gritted teeth, raging dizziness and waves of sadness, was a headache. A massive headache. *How had I not noticed all this pain?* I thought I had but really I'd just been ignoring it. Flirting round the edges of it, trying to deny its existence.

Headache

There must be a better word for this. Headaches come and go. We get them with colds and flus, we get them if we haven't been drinking enough and when we have drunk too much. They can last an hour or two, sometimes a day or two if it is a bad cold. Painkillers will help, they might not remove the pain completely but they do help.

This was like no headache I'd ever had before. And it went on for nearly a year. On a good day it was a throbbing ache, a drumbeat of pain in my skull. A background against which, with effort, I could almost think and life could carry on. If I could take frequent breaks, I was almost able to read. In the early months I had very few good days.

On bad days the throbbing ache was still there, but it was stronger, demanding my attention. Perhaps it felt outdone by the added sensation of a knife stabbing behind my left eye. Stabbing treble of pain at the front of my head, an answering bass of agony from the back. It was relentless and could go on for weeks without pause. Days were a ceaseless round of misery interspersed with attempts to eat and speak. I was gritting my teeth so hard against the pain that I cracked the molars again. But there was already so much going on that I didn't notice them aching too.

The hospital had sent me home with over-the-counter painkillers. Once the prescription ended, I bought more and used them every day. Paracetamol, ibuprofen, cold and flu preparations *What is phenylephrine? Who cares, it might help*. Nothing did. The bad days seemed endless and yet the world flew on without me.

Hallucinations

I waited in desperate faith that these symptoms would fade but there was no promised respite. Instead something else was going on which, when I realised the extent of it, would deeply affect my sense of self. It started with the phone ringing, or rather not ringing. After forcing myself awake from a nap I'd pick up the phone only to find it blank and asleep. No one had called, I'd just imagined it. The same would happen with text and email notifications, I'd even hear the doorbell go off with no one there.

Odd things were happening with my vision too, I was used to objects in my sight wavering to the left and snapping back, they'd been doing that for weeks. Once the spinning became familiar, I noticed 'sparkles' like mini fireworks going off in front of whatever I was looking at. It might have been entertaining, if it hadn't been so worrying. The real fear came from the periphery of my vision. There, the shadows would dart across the room. It would only be a matter of seconds for reality to reassert itself but the anxious heartbeat would take far longer to recover.

These hallucinations were terrifying. If you can't trust what you see and hear what can you trust? At the same time, my balance problems meant I felt I was about to fall off pavements into traffic. The fear became all consuming. After weeks feeling this terrified and vulnerable, I had shrunk. I crept along the edges of rooms, hugged close to buildings and tried to make myself as small as possible in public. Eventually, I just avoided leaving the flat altogether.

Daydreams and fantasy worlds

Human beings are social animals: we need the daily contact of other people. I was falling into a groundhog day of the same thing over and over again. I'd linger beside the door, waiting for the clang of the letterbox so

I could dash out in time to say good morning. The postman must have thought I was crazy. I was a strange woman he smiled at briefly once a day. He was the only person I'd see for hours while my husband was at work. Once he had gone there was little else to do. Reading books, listening to music or watching television all enraged the terrible headaches and nausea. Cognitive rest really meant doing nothing at all.

It is amazing what the brain can do to protect us. This world was no longer safe for me so my brain made a new one. It invented a place where I was away from pain and fear. A daydream world where I lived exciting lives with favourite characters from books or movies. In that made up world I was finally safe and I loved going there as the boring hours stretched out. But it also alarmed me. *Is this it? Is this how you lose your mind?*

Looking back, perhaps it was just my brain's way of keeping me entertained while it tried to heal. A neurological equivalent of 'We hope to resume normal service as soon as possible, meanwhile please enjoy our selected broadcast.'

The propensity to daydream faded over time. Though it still comes back whenever I've overdone it. When I'm exhausted and the cognitive fatigue means I need to lie still, not sleeping just resting, for hours on end. When the sheer boredom of doing nothing threatens to undo all of my precious recovery. It's then that the imagination comes to the rescue, giving me something to focus on and think about when nothing else is possible.

Desperate for more help I called the helpline of a brain injury charity, Headway, which my GP had mentioned. The call was answered by a trained nurse who had worked in A&E and head trauma for years. It was the first time someone had been able to relate to what I was going through, ask knowledgeable questions and provide much needed reassurance.

It seemed my experiences were following a pretty normal line for this type of injury. All this vague and incorrect information with wrong turns and false starts was par for the course for people with brain injuries. I was only just dipping a toe into the looking glass world of a 'brain injury survivor'. The phone call was helpful but there were a lot of acronyms to learn:

ABI = acquired brain injury.

This is an injury caused to the brain after birth and may be caused by external forces like a fall or an accident or by something internal, like a tumour or stroke.

TBI = traumatic brain injury.

An injury to the brain caused by a head injury. Is also an ABI.

PTA = post-traumatic amnesia.

This is a period of time after a head injury when someone may be confused. It doesn't just refer to how long someone can't remember things for, but might also mean that the person isn't aware of things around them or is behaving in an odd manner.

The relief I felt after receiving answers during that call spurred me on for more. I spent my lucid hours scavenging for information on websites, waiting room leaflets and charity pamphlets. I leaned that the severity of a TBI tends to be classified both by how long the person is unconscious and how long any PTA lasts. So, someone for whom PTA lasts more than 7 days, or who was unconscious for 48 hours would be classified as having a very severe brain injury.

I didn't lose consciousness and didn't seem to have much PTA so that meant I was in the 'mild' category. The strangest thing I learned was that there is such a thing as a mild traumatic brain injury. The very definition of an oxymoron.

Ok, confirmation that this is mildly traumatic. Any other gems can I unearth?

There were. A mild TBI is often caused by something hitting the brain or causing the brain to move inside the skull. An example might be when your car is rear-ended or, in my case, a shoulder barge to the face. Then there are often complications that follow this initial impact. So it was helpful to think of a TBI as a series of injuries.

A series of injuries in TBI

1. An impact or sudden movement means the head is rocked back and forth or rotated quickly which means the brain will move at speed too. This movement can twist, stretch or even break some of the brain's blood vessels, nerve fibres and connections. Also, the front of the skull often has sharp ridges and when the brain hits these it can cause more damage.
2. If the brain is not able to get enough oxygen, then any damage caused by the first injury will be exacerbated. This might happen if someone can't breathe because they are choking or if they are losing blood. Anything which interrupts the flow of oxygen rich blood to the brain in the seconds or minutes after the first injury could cause further problems.

3. The first two injuries tend to happen very quickly after an impact. The third injury may occur at the same time or it could happen days, even weeks later. This injury is caused by bleeding, bruising or swelling in the brain as it reacts to the damage caused by the initial impact.

Let's take my mild traumatic brain injury as an example. But do note that it is just my speculation. There was no clinical monitoring at the time nor in the months afterwards which could confirm any of this.

1. I was jumping forwards when the injury happened. The striker leapt into me so when her shoulder slammed into my nose, my head had been moving forward but was then snapped back. My brain continued moving forward and collided with the sharp ridges on the inside of my skull which had just been knocked backwards. As the forces reverberated, my brain then rebounded backwards and collided with the back of my skull. This was the first injury, the rocking of the brain inside the skull tearing or breaking the blood vessels and nerve fibres.
2. I was able to land on my feet before crumpling to my knees meaning there was fortunately no secondary impact of the head on the ground. As I was crouched forward, the blood poured out of my nose rather than going down my throat and I didn't choke. For this reason, and because I didn't lose consciousness, I was able to keep breathing. As a result, there was not a significant loss of oxygen to the brain, but there was still some loss. The blood now soaking into the grass was no longer delivering oxygen to my brain. And any blood leaking from the capillaries inside my brain was no longer delivering oxygen either. So, while the impact of a secondary oxygen starvation injury was not a primary factor in my resulting condition, neither was it a negligible one.
3. It would be a sensible bet that the third injury, the swelling injury, occurred between 24 and 36 hours after the initial impact. That is when the worst of my symptoms appeared, almost certainly exacerbated by a few glasses of wine that evening. However, this is all guess work, the x-ray taken at the first A&E department didn't pick up a broken nose and would have been completely incapable of picking up the swelling.

Three injuries then, not just one. It was oddly reassuring that there was more going on than I'd been told. At least there was a reason, no three reasons, as to why I felt like this. *What did my clinic notes actually say? Concussion, that was it. Search for that.*

Minor head injury aka concussion

This is a common form of mild TBI and is often caused by falls, road crashes, assault or sport accidents.

Bingo!

The symptoms include:

- confusion
- dizziness
- nausea
- headache
- problems with vision

Yep, these sound familiar.

There can also be memory problems and extreme fatigue. The symptoms of mild TBI do not seem mild to the person concerned.

No sh*t Sherlock!

Prolonged symptoms can lead to anxiety and depression.

Huh, no one mentioned that before.

When symptoms of a concussion persist, they are often called post-concussion syndrome.

Ah ha, there's that phrase again.

Generally, the vast majority of people with post-concussion syndrome make a full recovery, usually after three or four months.

Hurray!

However, there is a very small subgroup whose recovery is not so good.

Oh.

Time

On my second visit to the hospital the specialist had made clear how important it was to rest. 'Immediately. Your brain needs to stop now so it can heal.' This sense of urgency was repeated by my GP, the nurse on the charity helpline, waiting room leaflets and in online sources. One line stuck in my mind.

Quote from Headway – The Brain Injury Association (www.headway.org.uk)

'The greatest visible progress does occur in the first six months or so post-injury.'

There it was, a six-month window for me to heal as much as possible. I was only a sixth of the way into that time period, but seemed to be getting worse all the time. Prior to the injury, there was never enough time. Now I had plenty of time, but it was running out fast. Minutes and hours stretched on in a dizzy merry-go-round of bed, fridge, sofa, back to bed. But the weeks flew past at terrifying speed toward the six-month deadline of healing. I was trying to follow the orders to rest but couldn't stop myself worrying. *If this is the time when I get better, then when will I start getting better? And what if I'm still like this after six months has passed?*

Email to an International Judging Competition

ME: I regret that I will not be able to take part in the judging in two weeks' time. I received a blow to the head in March and my doctor has extended my time off work. I am very sorry for the late notice and hope you will consider me for the panel next year.

Despite the anxiety, I had to hope that I would be well enough to judge sake and wine again after twelve months. After all, if my post-concussion syndrome followed the most likely recovery curve, these symptoms would only hang around another week or two, right?

Right?

Reference

Headway – The Brain Injury Association (2014). Rehabilitation after brain injury. www.headway.org.uk. Available at https://www.headway.org.uk/about-brain-injury/individuals/rehabilitation-and-continuing-care/rehabilitation/ Last accessed May 2020.

Chapter 3

Abandonment and support

May: Two months after the incident

The response from Alder and my employer had been a huge relief. The response from my football team was a complete contrast. I had been with City United through several club transformations over 10 years and had taken various volunteer roles to help keep it going. At the time of the incident, my role was General Secretary, which meant I was responsible for keeping the club compliant with League rules. The medical advice meant I could no longer do this, and there was much to hand over. Immediately after the injury, I had tried to do just that.

Email sent to City United

ME: Hi Folks, think you all know I got a shoulder in the face at our last game. Turns out A&E got it wrong initially. My nose is broken but worse is the nasty concussion that will hang around for a few months.

The concussion is horrible, with a constant, awful dizziness. Recovery is a frustrating, unpredictable process and I can't do much at all. The phrase 'nasal deformity' was also used, which is hardly encouraging. Don't mind if nose sets wonky provided that I have a decent sense of smell when it does. Otherwise, might need a new career!

But priority is ensuring the brain heals. Doc says now that the recovery is all about doing nothing. I'm off work and cancelled everything so am not able to do the General Secretary role, please can you guys help?

I then spent more of my precious, dwindling brain power on a further page of specific instructions on what needed doing. This plea received just two replies which boiled down to 'That's awful but I'm too busy to help.'

The lack of empathy and refusal to respond, let alone help, had been devastating. *I thought they were my friends?!* Days later, the silence from City United was broken by an email asking me to help with the role, despite my previous explanation. I spent that day cobbling together a reply between naps and painkillers.

I tried, really tried to rest. But still felt a loyalty to my friends. It was something my husband didn't understand and, in hindsight, he was right. Why did I feel the need to help people who had ignored my situation and pleas for help? It made both my brain and heart ache.

Not everyone disappeared, though. One teammate had left in the off season for an overseas secondment and was unaware of what had happened to me. She had also spent months trying to hand over her former club duties and contacted me for help.

Summary of emails with Rowan

ME: (I filled her in on what had happened then…) After drooling on the sofa for six weeks I've have just been signed off to return to the office for 2 hours a day. Even this small amount is progress. Work have been very understanding but sadly this has put paid to my International Competition judging and the trade show at Caesars Palace. No Vegas for me!

Afraid that I've heard very little from anyone at City United in this time so can't answer your questions about the club's finances and treasury situation. However, I'll keep following you on social media and hope to see you when you return. Have a fantastic time out there.

ROWAN: God, I'm so sorry, that sounds awful. Is there scope for claiming under City United's insurance policy? Do you want me to look into it? I'll follow up the treasury stuff with the captain, no worries. Hope the concussion conks off sharpish.

Receiving that simple reply on my birthday meant a great deal to me, so much that I burst into tears. Rowan was on the other side of the planet and still found a way to help. It turned out that, while City United did have insurance, the policy didn't cover head injuries short of losing an eye or being in a coma – basically, 'show me the injury then I'll pay you'. This was my first tumble into one of the many loopholes around a hidden injury.

By this point you are probably thinking 'where on earth are her family?' My husband had been patient and supportive, amazing given how petulant, anxious, stressed and depressed I was. He responded to my fears with sensible logic that kept me calm and he never failed to tuck me in for the endless naps and sleep I needed. Ash had gone from having a loving, helpful partner in daily life to dealing with a confused, adult sized toddler who could barely think for herself.

My brother had followed us to London and now lived nearby. He had been an invaluable support given his previous, unrelated, experience with brain injury. My sisters were both down under so could not help beyond odd messages when the time difference allowed. However, my parents did not yet know there was a problem.

Just before the incident they had left New Zealand for a lengthy cruise across the Atlantic and around the Mediterranean. As they had been mostly incommunicado for that time, I hadn't wanted to worry them. Ash and I were to join them in Italy, the holiday, flights, and accommodation had been booked months before the incident.

The medical advice had assured us that I would be recovered for the holiday; after all, the initial prescription had been to 'take a week off football.' We also hoped that a change of scenery might help with my recovery. Plus, I wanted to see my mum.

The relief of a parent's hug after months of struggle and uncertainty made my knees buckle. I was a child again, wanting only to curl up in their arms until everything was ok. They knew something was wrong before I told them, of course they did! They are my parents and both trained medical professionals to boot. Given this and their past experience with another brain injury in the family they quickly stated something which I hadn't yet admitted to myself.

'You have to stop playing football.'

'What!?' *No, this is my thing. I'm a wine expert and footballer; it's my niche. It's me! What would I be if I can't be that anymore?*

At some point on the Amalfi coast I realised they were right. I was in one of the most beautiful places in the world, tearing round a hairpin curve on a bus which was an exhilarating roller coaster ride for everyone else. I was concentrating on trying not to pass out from dizziness and double vision. *I never want to feel like this again.*

I remember very little of a holiday which had been planned and anticipated for over a year. This holiday was filled with anxiety, tears and naps. But there were bright gems in there too: eating extravagant ice-creams in St Mark's square; lazy brunches while counting passing gondolas. These memories are glorious, I wish I could remember more.

Email to parents after the holiday

ME: Yep, went to the doctor's three days ago as planned. My GP knows as much about the recovery as I do. The hospital letters to her say less than I'm told in the appointments, at least, less than I can remember from the appointments. We agreed to trying half days of work again. I'm signed off on those for the next two weeks to see how it goes. I was in the office for half a day and am exhausted tonight. Everywhere I turned people were there asking how I am or needing decisions made. It will change as most people haven't seen me in weeks.

From my colleagues' point of view, my ten-week absence and gradual return was hard to understand. I hadn't been admitted to a hospital and, once the bruises on the face healed, I looked completely normal.

People react differently when told a colleague has had a car accident or a stroke, to being told they got a concussion playing football. Of course we do: look at how head injuries are treated in movies. Someone gets knocked out but leaps up again to go and save the world with a heroic act. There is seldom any memory loss and certainly no lasting impairment. I didn't even get knocked out, so why had I disappeared for so long and left them to take up the slack?

No one ever said this to me of course, and they probably didn't even think it. But I did. Turns out enhanced anxiety levels are a key indicator of a brain injury and a massive hindrance to the rest prescribed for recovery.

The return to work was a struggle, I was doing nothing but sleeping, eating and trying to work. One day I was forcing myself on a route march to the station, determined to make it in to the office. I was chanting 'take it easy' over and over, a mantra that might keep me calm. I spotted the early roses on a bush and in a fit of excitement decided to smell them. *Everyone should take time to smell the roses, keep the anxiety at bay, relax and feel fine.*

It didn't work. The scent exploded in my brain, exacerbated the whirling dizziness and sent panic flooding over fragile, barely coping bulwarks. Stopping to smell the roses sent me back to bed.

Numerous social events were missed: birthdays; weekends away; engagement parties; baby showers; weddings… I disappeared from the daily life of many of my friends. A few understood and hung around. Others dropped contact immediately or drifted away over time.

June: Three months after the incident

My mother had suggested keeping a diary, both as a memory aid and as proof of my slow recovery. Evidence which would provide solace on those days when everything was misery. The first week of entries focused on work. That seems odd but it was important. I felt that if I could get daily life back to normal then everything else would follow.

Diary entries

MONDAY: GP visit in the morning and then worked 3 hours in 30 min blocks at home.

TUESDAY: In office at 10 but pretty constant until 3.30 – not good.

WEDNESDAY: Worked at home, very quiet but not a good head day.

THURSDAY: (no entry)

FRIDAY: Two hours at home then tried to go to work, failed so nap & another hour of work at home.

WEEKEND: Quiet, head sore, a very slow weekend. But sorted footy.

Email to City United

ME: Please excuse the mass email, but it's been ages since I've been able to see anyone. I've tried to keep in touch but my life since March has been recovering from that blow on the nose I got against Anonymous FC. It was a long time ago but I still have ongoing problems. As well as a broken nose, I still have a nasty concussion that has had me drooling on the sofa for months. Good news is that I have just had my first week back at work, albeit part-time.

However, I can't play football again. I'm pretty gutted but the doctors say I've had too many knocks to the head and just can't risk another one. So that is a quarter of a century of footy over, along with most other sports I've enjoyed. Thank you to everyone for a great decade or so with the club; hopefully I can say these things properly over a pint some time. With any luck I'll be fit enough be a sideline stalwart when the new season starts but hope to see you all sooner than that. Please keep in touch!

This email gathered quite a few replies, though also notable silences. People I thought were good friends maintained their radio silence. The replies also revealed that many teammates had been unaware of what had happened. Those 'good' friends who had known the extent of my injuries hadn't passed the message on so most at City United thought I had simply disappeared.

It was then that I began doubting my own judgement. People I had assumed were friends abandoned me. News of my injury hadn't been passed on. My solid foundation of twenty-five years as a footballer was over.

Tweet

Three months after that blow to the head at footy & finally managed a week back at work. Only half days and am exhausted, but hurray! Progress!

That weekend, after struggling to complete four hours' work per day, I retreated to bed, a ball of anxious tears, pain and exhaustion. My confusion and frustration were all-consuming. I was told this would fix itself in a week, then it should be sorted in six weeks. Then it was a post-concussion syndrome that should go soon but might hang around for a year. *What have I done wrong? Had the doctors missed more than my broken bones?* By following the initial, ultimately erroneous, advice has further damage been caused?

Another trip to the GP ended in another sick note and more days off work. She noted that in pushing to get back to normal I was exhausting myself. The fatigue meant that the attempt at a diary ended. I would pick it up again in September, but the intervening three months are greyed out, with odd punctuation marks of memories.

July: Four months after the incident

Summary of emails with Hazel, a former teammate

HAZEL: Hey, how's things? Really hope you're feeling a bit better. Just have a question/invitation for you. I've been asked by River FC to start up a women's team. Now I know you can't play, but I wondered if you would want to be involved in a non- playing capacity anyway. To be clear I'm definitely not looking at trying to poach anyone from City United. This is totally independent of them. I could really do with a bit of a hand as starting up a team from scratch is a big job, but I'd also like some good mates involved. Much more fun that way. If you are tiny bit interested, whoop! Or feel free to tell me to bugger off.

ME: Good to hear from you! Yes, I'm interested so please send me over the proposal. Bear with me though, as there will be a definite limit to what I can do and my involvement would have to pause whenever I push it too much (that happens a lot!). In terms of our old team, yes, I too would want to be careful with how the new River FC team is presented. Afraid I can't tell you any more about feelings in City United since my injury. As the difficult weeks have worn on, I've heard very little from anyone. Suffice to say I woke up happy this morning for the first time in ages and am thinking of who me might contact to get the team started. So hope you'll take me on. Cheers and thanks for thinking of me.

I was ecstatic! *Perhaps my social isolation is coming to an end?* Months had gone by with little help from my friends at City United. But I was still the main contact listed with the FA and on the team's webpage. League administration and queries from new players demanded my limited attention. I dutifully sent these on to the team along with repeated requests to change contact details and the website. There was no reply and I continued to receive queries from the league and new players.

The silence was filled with loneliness and mood swings. I flew into rage or despair at any evidence of other people getting on with their lives while I was stuck in endless days of nauseous pain and fatigue. I wanted to scream: *What about me?* We were friends, we cried and laughed together through your break ups and your triumphs. *Where are you now that my world has fallen apart?*

Fortunately, anaesthesia for the brain came along in the form of the Football World Cup. I vaguely remember watching games, though it would be more accurate to say that I sat on the sofa and drooled at the screen. I didn't enjoy the tournament, fast moving images meant following the action was beyond my comprehension. But I used to like watching football so perhaps, if I made myself do things that I normally did then I'll get back to normal?

The rest of July flew past. Despite the time that had passed since the incident I don't have many memories of what happened. And plenty happened. We were helping friends with organising their wedding at the end of the month, I was trying to fulfil three half days at work per week and doing what I could behind the scenes to set up a new team with River FC. From the emails and scraps of memories that remain, it seems the month went like this:

- Hen and birthday parties, missed.
- Shopping trips, compulsory. *I can't go to a wedding in my pyjamas.*
- Feathers to ruffle or soothe alternately, mostly mine.
- Meetings for work or River FC, missed.

Fortunately, I do retain a few memories of the wedding. The most treasured is hugging my husband while we watched our friends' first dance. As they shimmered in sequinned happiness everything seemed just fine.

August: Five months after the incident

Meanwhile, as if I didn't have enough sh*t going on, things had really kicked off with the football teams. *Pardon the pun, I just had to.* As the new season was approaching, Hazel and I decided it would be best for City United to find out about the River FC team from us. We knew there would be questions and wanted to keep things friendly, or at least civil. Hazel sent City United a friendly email and I followed up.

Summary of emails with City United

ME: Howdy folks, just to let you know I'm working with River FC on setting up the new team. I'd hoped to meet to talk to you all in person, but perhaps you'd like to arrange that meet up soon? Hope the summer training in this heat is going ok.

CITY UNITED COACH: Thanks for your email. Would you not prefer to help advance our team and help to recruit new players for us? As you know, there are loads of things involved with running a football club, plus things that we never get to do because everyone's so busy: Like getting a better training pitch, having a proper website… I just thought that you would rather be part of that than in setting up a rival team.

When the email popped up, I was thrilled. *They've replied, at last!* But I was, perhaps naively, stung by being called a rival. And I had already been doing a lot of those neglected tasks for City United before the incident. This long-awaited reply seemed to say 'Why don't you keep doing all the stuff that we never really thanked you for while we play the football that you can't enjoy anymore?'

Maybe this is unfair, but my diplomacy was strained from months of pain and loneliness. I managed to reply with:

ME: Basically, I'm involved with River FC because they got in touch. I've been trying to meet with you guys to talk about this but had no replies. To what extent I can be involved with either team I don't know. Sadly, it is one of the many things dependent on a recovery that no one can predict. Ultimately, I was contacted by a friend asking for help that

I was both able and excited to give. So, I will be helping her when I can, though advice is really all I'm fit for at moment. I'd be happy to help you guys too, but if working with River FC means you see me as a rival will that work? I'd still like to meet up with you guys for a pint and to discuss face to face please?

There was no reply. Unless you count the rumours. It's fairly impressive that I heard them at all, given my social isolation. They must have been widely shared and the few that got back to me were both unpleasant and untrue. I had been ignored long before Hazel got in touch, but now there was an excuse. Something to let City United off the hook for abandoning a friend.

I'd like to say I drew a line under this. That I dropped my feelings of hate, abandonment and sadness. That I wrote it off as a lesson to be learned and just enjoyed the memories of our fantastic friendships.

But I'd be lying. I cried for days on end and questioned my judgement for ever considering them friends. My former teammates were tried in the court room of my feelings and, in my time of greatest need, found wanting again and again. 'Ghost' is an awful term which just makes one feel transparent, diluted by pain and anguish.

One day, after weeks of doubt and rage, I decided I couldn't cry about them anymore. It was hard, but I moved on. I'd been shown how by some incredible friends who deserved far more attention than I'd been giving them.

People fall in and out of sports and hobbies all the time, so what made this team so special? They were the team that brought me friends when I'd first arrived in London. I had given a lot to the club, and over the years had undertaken nearly every volunteer management role going. But once the other managers found I couldn't play football anymore most of them stopped speaking to me. Well, I wasn't the first person City United had done this to. In fact, I'd previously behaved just like those people I now vilified. Nothing teaches humility like walking in the footsteps of those you have persecuted. I swallowed my hypocrisy and sat down at the keyboard.

Summary of emails with Maple, a former teammate whom I had excluded

ME: I'm really sorry I've not been in touch since the Halloween party, can't believe it was that long! But I do know that I had a night… well… unlike any since I was at University. So, if I did anything to offend, please be assured I didn't mean it and I apologise profusely! I am also writing because we are setting up a ladies' team with River FC. Would you be interested in returning to football? Please let me know if you are or if you would like to meet for a catch up as it would be great to see you.

MAPLE: Thank you for writing. It has been a while and I have been thinking about you. I heard about your injury and hope you are ok. Don't worry about the Halloween night. Many people said many hurtful things so I distanced myself from City United. I am really glad that the River FC team is happening. Would love to meet up and catch up about that and how you are doing. Let me know when you are free.

Now that's how to forgive gracefully: an example I desperately needed. We had lunch that week. The resurrection of a friendship is a precious thing, and thinking of Maple always makes me smile.

I saw Maple and several other friends at the end of that month. Hazel and I had organised a five-a-side tournament to advertise River FC and, hopefully, attract new players. The long day meant I pushed through my fatigue and dizziness. Apparently, I was on the ball, helping to run the tournament and didn't tune out once. But I don't really remember as, yet again, I paid in lost memories. There are a few moments which I hug close. A beautiful late summer day full of laughter, friendly competition and good-natured ribbing.

The brain suffered badly afterward, my dizziness and headache were back to their worst levels. It took a week of sleeping and doing nothing before I could contemplate leaving the house again. My mental state during that week was terrible as I struggled with pain and fear. The six-month 'window of healing' was over, and I still suffered for days after only a few hours of normality. Recovery was horribly slow.

Chapter 4

Returning to normal after brain injury

Life gets in the way

September: Six months after the incident

A milestone, a time to draw a line under things and move on. It was in this frame of mind that I woke up on a day off and set up a lunch date with Laurel. Time to haul my ass out of self-pity and get on with things. If I could manage that, maybe the recovery will follow.

Then I saw the email from my parents in New Zealand. My sister had been admitted to hospital with chest pains and, given the time difference, they hadn't wanted to wake us up so sent an email. Naturally I called them straight away, but I don't remember doing so. Once again it is emails that tell me what happened.

Those messages to friends and the wider family reveal that I was tempted to fly to New Zealand immediately. But, even if I'd raced to Heathrow and managed to get the first flight home, it would still be two days before I arrived. All we could do was wait and see how things were in twelve hours. So, I had a cuppa and thought about leaving the house.

'Seriously, you just had a cup of tea?' Laurel was alarmed by the morning's news.

'What else am I supposed to do? My sister is safely in hospital. My parents could be there in a few hours if needed but we are all waiting to see what the evening brings. Or rather what the morning brings. It is night there and day here so they're trying to sleep while we're trying to eat.'

'Fair enough, distance means there is little you can do. How are you?'

'Urgh, struggling. I keep trying to get back to normal but everything is just dizzy and awful. I feel like sh*t the whole time but being in the house just makes me feel trapped. Meanwhile most of my football friends are shunning me, my career and hopes of being a director are down the toilet and I struggle to just shower.'

'Forget about work. I know you've been off for a while but you'll pick things back up again. Right now, it's just something you shouldn't be worrying about. Lots of woman take months off and still get their career back on track. Ok, you didn't plan this time off and it isn't for maternity reasons, but there's no reason you can't do the same.'

'You're right. I woke up trying to be positive this morning. Every now and then I feel like I'm getting on top of things only for something else to happen. But all I'm talking about is me, I'm just self-centred at the moment. What are you up to?'

Laurel's pep talk helped, as did getting out of the house and hearing about other people's lives for once. I'd been wrapped up in my own life and had been in a frame of mind where news of other people gave me a horrible sense of missing out. Depression means you focus on the negative ahead of the positive. Witness all that time I'd spent agonising over the friends who had dropped me and not thought about those who had stood by me, or returned to help in the last few months. *But, as of today, things will be different!*

On the bus home after lunch, I was drained. The fight against dizziness and nausea was constant, but I was happy. My life felt more balanced than it had been over the last few months. I needed ear plugs to dull sound and dark sunglasses to hide behind but had managed to reach a small place where I could smile despite the pain. As I walked home from the bus stop, I sent Laurel a message with thanks for a lovely lunch.

Suddenly, the phone was gone. It was wrenched from my hand by a boy who had ridden his bike onto the pavement. Just like in a classic horror movie it came when I least expected it. The punk with my phone bounced his bike back onto the road and raced off to the cheers of his accomplices. Instinct kicked in and I sprinted after them shouting that terrible cliche 'Stop! Thief!'

Huh, people really do say that.

Another part of me thought: *Like this is going to work.*

Shut up, and just run!

One block later the cycle gang and my phone were still in sight but my legs and lungs burned from the unaccustomed effort. I came to a hopeless stop and a passer-by said:

'Like that is going to work.'

Huh, told you.

'Just call the police.'

'I can't, they got my phone.'

'Oh, I'll call them now for you.'

As he dialled, another neighbour raced past on a mobility scooter. The engines revved as he cried out 'I'm after them!' Then he hunkered down behind the plastic windshield. The chase was on!

The police were there quickly, within five minutes. While my knight on trusty mobility steed hadn't yet returned, a local lad had turned up. He'd seen what had happened and knew the gang from school. It turns out the police also knew them. The scootered vigilante reported in. He had followed the group through several council estates before losing them. I was barely keeping track of events, struggling to process simple sentences through the dizziness. That was clear to the officers.

'Have you taken anything today? Anything that might be making you sway a bit?'

'What? No, it's all just a bit overwhelming.'

They continued assessing me before I finally twigged.

'No, I'm not on anything, I'm off work recovering from a head injury.'

Their faces changed, more sympathetic but also tense. They knew how to deal with drink and drugs, how did you handle someone who just 'wasn't right in the head'? We sat on a bench, and they went through it slowly for me.

'Ok, your other device can't track your phone which means they've shut it down completely. So, we can't track it but your data is safe. We'll follow up at their homes but they won't go there with a stolen phone. They'll take it straight to a shop, wipe it and sell it on. It'll be overseas within a week.'

'So how will I get it back?'

'Your phone is gone. That's the most likely scenario. When you get home, you can use the security apps to erase your data remotely when it is next turned on.'

'So that will be ok, but why can't I get my phone back if you know who has it?'

'Like I said they'll sell it straight away, probably already have. We'll follow up at their addresses but they won't have it.'

'But my sister has been admitted to hospital in New Zealand, I need to know how she is. I need my phone.'

'I'm sorry, but your phone is gone.'

They were patient with me and called back the next day with an update. Sure enough, there was no evidence of the phone at any of the perps' homes. I could try to press charges over the act of theft without physical evidence. That would mean the young lad who witnessed the theft would need to testify. He wanted to, but the gang knew him so his parents were worried about bullying, or worse. By this time, Ash had helped me to understand what had happened and we'd discussed this possibility.

'No, I won't press charges. The phone is gone and I'm not going to ask a kid to go through that. Please thank him for wanting to do the right thing.'

'Sorry about this, it's the first phone snatch we know of round there.'

'There's a first I could do without. Still I got to shout "Stop Thief" so at least that's something out of the day.'

'A life ambition realised. Um, how's your sister?'

'Thank you, she is back home now after quite a scare, but on the mend.'

We signed off and I went for a desperately needed nap. Little did I know I'd be calling the police twice more in the next year.

Email to self

List of tasks:

- Make sure all doctor appointments are in the diary
- Check Police report is accurate
- Tell Hazel can't make new training dates
- Make sure eye test is in diary. Remember to tell them about the double vision and spots. Also concussion
- Schedule all meetings for morning where possible
- Schedule one day working from home every week
- Amend employer's meeting minutes as per attached
- Copy finalised spreadsheet into report and distribute

I often lay awake at night panicking about the things I might forget. The coping mechanism was to email myself a list. It usually worked and meant I could sleep without struggling to remember what I'd decided to do. It also led to jumbled, repetitive lists, but it worked for me.

Every day was filled with the hope that something would click and my life would return to normal. The world had turned upside down in an instant, was it so much to ask that it would sort itself out as quickly too? I was determined to get back to normal so when the time came for the next sick note, I agreed to try five half-days per week. On the basis of what we knew of the injury, it seemed like the next thing to do.

It didn't work, and in the middle of the office, I collapsed again in spectacular fashion. Alder walked me to the train station, somehow putting one foot after the other while my fear and neurosis broke around him.

'In all seriousness, may I suggest counselling? Sometimes just the power of speaking to someone, saying things to an objective person who isn't involved, can be very healing.'

It was very sensible advice, but when do we ever listen to sense? Plus, I had a career to rebuild, a hen party to get to and a football team to construct. Life doesn't just stop because your brain needs too.

But my brain did stop. And it was stopping for longer than I realised at first. Hours would pass as I stared at nothing. Brain and body as flat as possible. I wasn't in there, not really. I was floating somewhere. Somewhere out there. Where amber and red leaves fluttered in the strong breeze.

When this headache started, the tree outside our bedroom was a stark silhouette. Bare branches in an early spring day. Now it shone in autumnal finery. Branches bedecked in gold and ruby stood out against a clear blue sky. It called like a beacon, urging movement and joy. A celebration of life.

The dizziness spins endlessly, fatigue pins me to the bed. I roll away from the window. The world rolls on without me.

Summary of emails with parents

MUM: We've been worried about your popping in and out of work. The stress of it seems to affect you at home, and your recovery. I was thinking about our family's attitude to work, not that it's actually done us badly in the long run. For our family, 'Work' has always been capitalised as it was the priority. We needed to get ready for it and be organised. Up, breakfast, out the door first thing and always early. So, I was amazed, quietly appalled, then realistic about the attitude of a few colleagues.

They would turn up at 9am and check the emails for anything urgent while eating breakfast. At 10.30 one would pop out to buy the lattes and then all would sit around for the morning tea and chat. Back to work for an hour or so then out to the gym, or shopping, hair, whatever. Lunch was consumed at the desk on their return and more work until the afternoon tea chat. Office was tidied and computers shut down early so they could leave at 5pm on the dot without taking any mental work thoughts with them. I have no doubt they worked hard and as part of the team. Work was a job, not a vocation and certainly not something to drag, cart or carry around. It was the way to pay bills and have a life, not something they were striving to achieve or improve.

It's not easy finding the mid-way between doing it well and having no anxiety. The knack, I think, is leaving it in the office. You remember our friend who was a social worker and commuted by ferry? Her habit was to throw things mentally overboard on the way home, and pick them up on the way back. I've not managed to off load work like that and nor did your father. Perhaps you can?

ME: Yes, it is something I think we have as a family but that doesn't mean it can't be beaten! Lots of people in my office are just like those in your email. Which I guess is why I get all the questions and time critical projects and they don't. It will be difficult to stop that trend, but if I can't say no when I'm recovering from a brain injury when can I?

Summary of emails with Hazel

HAZEL: Just done an attendance list for the four training sessions we've held. Those sessions have drawn in thirty-four people and twenty-one who want to play at our first game. Hope you're feeling a bit better – just thought I'd share the good news!

ME: Wow, that's great news. Well done! Building a team from scratch is not an easy thing to do. I am pottering on. The age-old problem of stress in the workplace is causing problems and am struggling with things that aren't really my job. So today was day one of saying 'No I can't, but I'm confident you could.' I managed a morning of it before the CEO had a word. He'd overheard me and wanted to check I was ok. Seems me saying 'No' to a task is unusual enough to be a concern!

Parties and irritability

At the end of the month I was invited to a hen party which I was determined to make. A full day of activities was planned from 10am until well into the wee hours. Normally I'd be one of the first to arrive and last to leave. Despite my insistence on being as normal as possible, I had to admit that a full day out was not going to happen. Looking at the events carefully, I figured I could manage the afternoon events: bowling followed by bingo, and cabaret hosted by a fabulous drag queen – sounds fun!

I didn't think about the practicality of someone battling severe dizziness issues putting on unfamiliar shoes and throwing around heavily weighted balls on a slippery surface. Fortunately, my friends stepped in and I was declared a spectator for the bowling. This proved to be a sensible suggestion as the attempt to get an alcohol-free beverage took all my concentration.

'Was that with vodka or gin?'

'Just a lime and soda please.'

'What with though?'

'No alcohol, just a lime and soda please.'

'What are you driving or something?'

'Something like that.'

After a dubious look the bartender filled the order and plonked the glass on the counter. 'Definitely no gin or vodka yeah?'

'Yeah.' I replied and handed over £10. The bar tender returned with a fiver.

'Hang on, where's the rest of it?'

'Well, that's £5.'

'For water and cordial?'

'Yeah, the till automatically charges for a shot of alcohol and I don't know how to do it otherwise.'

The bar was empty except for me, but the wait for the manager dragged on. When the manager finally arrived, she split her time between polishing glasses and giving me disgusted looks while the server explained the situation. I missed much of the bowling. In the end I got my tenner back and they kept the now flat water.

The injustice of this sat with me right through to the drag queen cabaret. Even singing 'Jerusalem' in a hot tent while doing the Hokey Cokey couldn't stop me from picking at it. I didn't know it at the time but I was exhibiting two more common side-effects of brain injury: irritability and obsessiveness. I couldn't let go of the fact that it proved so hard to get a decently priced alcohol-free drink.

This mingled with my need for control and I resolved to speak out at the next injustice that I saw. I didn't have to wait long. When the hen won a bingo line but wasn't the first to call out, I protested loudly to the whole audience.

'Why doesn't my friend get a prize too? It's just unfair that everyone with a bingo line doesn't share equally.'

Laurel was there, and averted a bigger scene by quietly calming me down. She took me outside and helped me get the train home.

Diary entry

SUNDAY: Big day – first game for the new River FC team. I managed to be out of the house for hours cheering people on or in a busy pub. Plus I navigated public transport there and back!

This note in my diary doesn't capture the feelings of being back on a football pitch for the first time since the incident. It was both familiar and threatening territory. I wasn't playing of course. My brief was to encourage the goal keeper, who was kept busy given this was the first time the defence had run together.

While I do have memories of this game, they are odd and slightly dissociated. I've never been afraid of the ball before, perhaps that is why I didn't recognise the small person hiding far behind the goal nets cringing at every shot? I'd been good enough to play in goal for a premier league reserve team so of course I wouldn't whimper when a wayward shot whizzed past metres away.

The excitement and anxiety of the football match led to two days of dizzy bed rest. Finally, I forced myself out of bed and out the door. The GP had emphasised the need to keep doing exercise to help the recovery. So I had my first walk outside in days. It really helped to clear the head but left me completely exhausted and with yet another lightheaded, dissociated feeling.

This was pretty much the pattern six months on from the incident. I needed at least twelve hours of sleep to be sure of enough energy for eating, work, exercising and getting more sleep. If I got this mix wrong, the consequences were nasty.

Despite my optimism at the start of the month, things hadn't just snapped back into place. I was a long way from normal and wasn't even sure I was on the right path. Was there really nothing more modern medicine could do for me? I phoned the brain charity helpline which had been so calm and reassuring when I'd last called. Following their advice, I emailed my GP.

Email to GP

ME: Thank you for the recommendation of the further counselling services, I have been in contact with them and am also going for an eye check-up today. I am writing to also ask for a referral onto a neurologist please? I've been speaking with the helpline you mentioned and they suggested that would be worth doing alongside the counselling services.

Tweet

When calling the NHS, you are asked to hold before being told to ring another number... which no-one ever answers. 40mins & 8 phone calls later I finally speak to a person who can help! Ah, she gave me another number where I can leave a message. Hurray?

Despite these problems, I did manage to confirm my appointment in the earliest available adult brain injury clinic. However, that was more than two months away, in December. Now it was just 'hurry up and wait.'

It had been a hell of a busy September. After a horrible six months I had managed to increase my work hours a little. But the month ended with another nasty relapse of neurological symptoms. So, I began October with:

- another three weeks signed off work
- an appointment for an MRI scan
- and appointment at an adult brain injury clinic

Best of all, I'd had reassurance that there was more which could be done.

Email to friends

ME: I've been doing it all wrong! Reports out today show that there is a flavonoid in beer which boosts brain power, and turmeric can help the brain to heal! You guys up for curry & beer sometime?

Chapter 5

Seeking professional help

Hard truths to face

October: Seven months after the incident

I really needed sleep, but it was still elusive. Even seven months on I was always dizzy. However still I lay, the bed felt like it was spinning in space. If I managed to ignore that then there was the ringing tinnitus to overcome, all mixed in with the anxiety of an insomniac for whom sleep is an unachievable aim.

The grey days of early autumn slipped past. In this half-life routine of trying to get 'normal', the days were often mixed up in my diary. The reward for these horrid weeks on the sofa was a pass from the GP to try another return to work. Her plan was to ease me back by trying three hours of work from home every day. It felt manageable. But I woke on the first day with a very dizzy headache after a night of broken sleep and a worrying throb at the site of the injury on my nose. I managed to do two days of work, then had the third off for a hospital visit.

First MRI scan

A poor night's sleep meant this whole day had a slow 'moving through treacle and dizzy fog' feeling. I took the bus to yet another hospital and reported for my first MRI. I was so pleased that at last we would be looking inside the mess of my brain that, when I was directed to a shipping container in the car park, I didn't bat an eyelid. Seems there wasn't room in the old Victorian building so this modern technology was allotted a disabled parking space at the extreme rear of the hospital grounds. In hindsight, it was hardly reassuring, but my poor scrambled braincells were just trying to get through the day so the odd setting barely registered.

Safety briefing ticked off, I was delivered into the magnet on a conveyor belt. *Fresh meat for the grinder.* Those really weren't the relaxing thoughts

I needed in order to stay still through the roaring and grinding of the scan unit. I'd been told this would take about half an hour and that some people slept through it. *Really?* If I can't sleep in the safety and peace of a warm bed, I'd never manage it here. *Breathe, concentrate on the breathing. Make sure you keep doing that, at least.* The words of the meditation lessons came back and I counted the breaths in and out while a whirring magnet tried to find the reason for the last seven months of pain. Finally, the scan was over.

'OK, you did very well. Head back out to the cloak room area and you can collect your things. Your GP will get a letter in a week or so.'

With impressive efficiency I was bundled back out into the light mist of October, clutching my belongings and straws of hope.

Diary entries

FRIDAY: I'm catching up in the diary even though the last two days have been empty and slow. I am exhausted and the dizziness is worse. Walking is an effort. I'm grasping furniture to avoid falling over again. It feels like I'm back to those first terrible weeks immediately after the incident. On both days I have needed sixteen hours of sleep and didn't manage to do any work at all. Finding it depressing to be so immobile but I do recognise the need to go to bed & sleep more. Hoping scan would help – but not sure how. The results are due Monday. But even if nothing shows up I still have a two month wait until the neurology clinic appointment.

MONDAY: An appointment with the nurse today for a flu vaccine. I was hoping that I would also get news on the MRI scan but those results aren't due for another four days. That shows how out of whack my sense of time is lately! The vaccination was over quickly but the nurse stretched the appointment out. She noticed the change in me since my last, pre-incident, visit and took the time to speak with me. It was a relief to talk with someone who was both objective and caring. The nurse said that the injury had obviously caused me to lose confidence in myself and that I needed counselling quite desperately. I told her about the long waiting list for the local NHS services and she mentioned a few private businesses. This was the third time that someone had mentioned counselling. Perhaps it is time to try it? The appointment turned out to be far more emotional than expected so left feeling quite drained. I managed to get a nap in before going to the dentist again. Hopefully that is the last of the repairs to the cracked molars. Quiet evening but need bed soon.

THURSDAY: The good news is that I managed to sort out an appointment with a local volunteer counselling service. And I managed to speak to GP surgery about the scan results. My normal GP was not available so I was put through to a colleague who intoned 'all it says here is "normal". Ho hum, still no answers. I see my GP for our regular back to work assessment on Monday so perhaps I'll get more information then. The work question will be important too. I have managed only two & a half hours work so far this week. My manager, Alder, needs to know the timescale for my return to work as he meets with the CEO again in a week. While I was talking to Ash about my fears over whether doing more work would help or hinder my recovery, I felt very unstable and dizzy.

Ash was having to deal with a few troubles at the moment. Alongside the struggle of living with an impaired wife, the company he contracted for hadn't paid him for months. He was already owed thousands in pay arrears before we discovered the company was being investigated by the tax man and had been telling the staff several 'mistruths'. Fortunately, we were able to manage financially as I was still on salaried sick leave and we had some savings. In between soothing me, Ash was exploring avenues to recover his pay and searching for new contracts.

It was the hottest and driest October since records began, but we'd not enjoyed it much. There was work going on at a neighbour's flat, so our outside space was full of scaffolding and builders for weeks. All in all, we needed a break so spent a warm Halloween visiting friends. It was nice to get out but the long day left me very dazed and exhausted. The weather wasn't the only thing out of sorts.

November: Eight months after the incident

Diary entry

SUNDAY: I seem to be over-sensitive to every little change in brain. Psycho-somatic? Fear & anxiety? Last night I had horrid dreams, keep waking & dozing.

The next day I woke anxious and jaded before my regular GP appointment. She wasn't able to expand on the results of the MRI scan.
'I'm sorry, we are just told that it looks normal.'
'But it isn't. It can't be. Please, I just want to be…normal again.'
'I know you want to get back to work but, you aren't well enough.'

'So what can I do to get well, what is the right answer?'

'At present, we have no answers, right or wrong. The ABI clinic in December might have some for us. We need to get you strong for that.'

'Yeah, makes sense.'

'Let's sign you off again, but this time until after you have seen the ABI clinic.'

'That's next month. You want to sign me off for a month-long leave of absence?'

'Yes, I think it is for the best.'

The appointment left me depressed. Each monthly anniversary of the incident would bring a burst of hope that this might be the time when I could be me again. Eight of these milestones stretched out behind me and I still struggled. I confess I cried myself into the afternoon nap.

The day had yet more in store as I had my first counselling session that evening. At first, I was hesitant. *How can I reveal myself to a complete stranger, when it's taking all my strength just to hold it together?*

Willow was careful to introduce herself and help me to feel safe. 'All that is in this room is you.'

Then she was quiet. It is true that if you leave a silence then the other person will feel the urge to fill it. And boy, did I fill it. Once the floodgates opened the worries of the last year came pouring out. I started with the incident of course, of the treatments and how they hadn't worked. Then fretted over the path of a career thrown off track, and the loss of my friends and the pain and tears. Back to the injury with more pain and tears. Then the fear that I'd always be a stumbling wreck of dizzy pain. I soaked through one tissue after another before shuddering to a halt. Willow had contributed only murmurs of solace and encouragement but now it was her turn to fill the room.

'That is overwhelming, I think anyone would be struggling with even half of that. When you say it out loud, a lot has happened.'

The relief of hearing someone assure you that it is ok to not be ok had me reaching for more tissues. As this round of tears dried Willow spoke again.

'In what you have said, and when I look at you, I see fear, sadness, anger, anxiety, depression and frustration mixed with a feeling of having no control anymore.'

'Yes! Yes, that all rings true. But why hadn't I noticed them, noticed those feelings?'

'Perhaps you have been clinging on to getting back to normal so hard that you haven't seen where you are now?'

'I've been so busy trying to get better.'

'That's understandable, you've been following what you've been told to do.'

'But it hasn't worked.'

'But you haven't given up and just sat on the couch. It's impressive to see that you are still fighting, that you clearly want more than this and want to work for it.'

Oh, that was so reassuring to hear. Yes, I am trying, bloody hard! 'But it is so tiring, I just… I just want to relax!'

'Maybe that is what you need just now. Relaxing isn't the same as resigning to this. It doesn't mean you are giving up. It just means you need a break right now.'

This time the tissue mopped up warm tears of relief. 'I needed that, I needed to hear it.'

Later that night, I updated the diary with the day's events and symptoms:

> Tired tonight, tinnitus and feeling nauseous again but head feels calmer, maybe?

I was booked to see Willow every Monday for the next six weeks. After the first session I was still not sure what good would come of it. But I couldn't deny the relief I'd felt while talking to someone who had no other involvement in my life. The calm I felt was brief as I began worrying about the reaction of my employer to the new, extended leave of absence. I needn't have feared as, just like with the initial sick notes, Alder took care of everything.

Summary of email from Alder

ME: It was good to speak with you last week and I'm pleased there are more possibilities for treatments now. As we discussed, we will need to arrange for a replacement for you, during this further leave of absence. Your team have done their best without you for the past eight months but they need clarity. I will meet with the CEO to discuss this.

We have now reached the point with your condition where the duration of your entitlement to full pay whilst absent on sick leave, under the terms of your contract, has been reached. We thus need to move on to a Statutory Sick Pay basis. This will be paid to you in exactly the same way as your salary through the monthly payroll and we will make the change on 1st December. In order for us to continue to pay you on this basis we simply need copies of your GP sick notes. We hope and expect as your condition improves that you will be able to resume working with us and we will make every effort to help you to manage your return to full fitness. Please let me know if you need any more information on this or if I can be of any help in any way.

Diary entry

MONDAY: I am dazed & drained after the second counselling session with Willow. We spoke about the fear I had in the early months and how I'd hidden it all. She showed me how guilty I'd been feeling. Guilt because there'd been no explanation as to why the symptoms had lasted so long. And yet at the same time a conflict because I didn't want people to worry about me. Teary & exhausted so off to bed feeling very dizzy & room spinning again.

December: Nine months after the incident

At one of my GP visits I weighed in at nearly 15kg (2st) overweight. I'd gone from two football sessions and 40miles of cycling every week to living on the sofa or in bed. I couldn't tell feelings apart any more so when the dizziness and nausea came, I didn't know if I was hungry, thirsty or tired. Even nine months on I didn't have the energy to work out which one it was. Inevitably, I went for the shotgun approach; have a snack, a drink and nap. My anxiety and depression demanded comfort food, which only added to the problem.

This combination did not lead to a healthy lifestyle, and my clothes agreed. One night I sat down and my trousers exploded. Diet was one of the few things I felt I might be able to get control of again. I tried for a day, then the brother intervened. 'You can't starve a brain injury! Sort this first and then worry.'

Tweet
Problem: I can't stop eating all the cookies!
Solution: Ate all the cookies

Email to Rose, a friend in the United States

ME: Winter has definitely started over here, the sun has set by 4pm and doesn't rise till nearly eight. I was out for a bit of shopping today and it was three degrees at 1pm. Actually, the weather is pretty much perfect for me as I have to plan my days carefully to avoid 'zonking out'. We've realised that for every two hours out and about with people I need a day in bed. Ho hum. My calendar is full of days blocked out so I might manage at least one Christmas party this year. Frustrating!

Clinic letter: Adult brain injury

> **Re: Appointment with ABI clinic:** We regret to inform you that
> your appointment has been cancelled. I apologise for the inconve-
> nience this may cause.

Diary entries

FRIDAY: After a decent morning, disaster struck when I checked the post. The letter said my appointment was cancelled. After months of wait-ing, it was a bitter disappointment. I broke down as I read it. Once I had control of myself, I picked up the phone. It took several hours of phone calls to find out what had happened. Turns out that the clinic my GP had booked all those weeks ago doesn't actually exist. Despite me calling to confirm the appointment, it took nine weeks to realise there was no clinic. They might be able book me an appointment with a specialist nurse in January but there are no neurologist appointments until February at the earliest now. I had to go bed & cry myself to sleep for a few hours. To be reduced to this, a grown woman crying at a cancelled appointment. But need to keep telling myself that this wasn't my fault and that there was nothing more I can do. Feel very dizzy & fragile this evening.

THURSDAY: Despite dropping off finally about 2am I slept soundly till 10 so managed eight hours uninterrupted sleep! Just need to move that eight hours to a more suitable time. Tried again to confirm the appointment with a specialist nurse now that my faith in the booking system has been severely rattled. That process proved stressful with yet more con-flicting information and another promise that they would call me back.

The brain charity helpline proved more useful, saying a diagnosis would probably say what we already know: a brain injury following accident. They suggested I try for referrals to help with the symptoms; so, a neuro-psychologist for my cognitive problems and a vestibular, or inner ear sys-tem, clinic to help with the balance. However, I found this advice difficult to accept. It felt like giving in, like admitting 'this can't be fixed, just man-age the symptoms'.

Definitely not what I want. I don't want to manage them, I want to get rid of them! So, I tried calling a private hospital. Apparently, someone calling up to pay privately rather than through insurance wasn't a common thing. My long phone call consisted of numerous transfers to the wrong departments. Ultimately, I was put through to a generic voicemail and cut off. Not promising!

Clinic letter: Adult brain injury

> We are pleased to confirm that a new appointment has been booked for you on January the 15th.

This letter appeared out of the blue, despite my frequent calls to the clinic. So, I called them up again, as all trust in the booking system had disappeared. The receptionist recognised my voice as I'd been calling so often. But they didn't know about this appointment and were also confused. It took another week for them to confirm the clinic actually existed and that I was booked into it.

Email to Rose

ME: Totally understand the bitter feelings of scrambling for treatment after the last few months. Crying myself into an afternoon nap is still my way of dealing with the struggle for answers. I am getting better on my own, slowly but surely. However, I still zone out when I try to do two things at once. We discovered today, when I broke down mid-conversation, that listening to someone speak while squeezing a tea bag counts as two things. I've been assured that all a specialist is likely to diagnose is 'brain damage following head injury' and then refer me on. Still, even that would be nice.

Diary entry

NEW YEAR'S EVE 2014: Well, 'Auld Lang Syne' takes on a bit of a new meaning this year. I'm not usually one for looking back in a maudlin way but… crikey!

It had been a roaring start to the year with days away on business. My employer had sent me to Japan in January and then to Beijing in February. I remember thinking Maldives in March, Las Vegas in April, can I be away on business every month this year? It certainly seemed possible with the required trips to Hong Kong in June, October & November and India on the cards at some point.

But what a difference one mis-timed leap by another person can cause! That striker has no idea of the damage she has done. Given the tough attitude of her team, and my goal saving tackles in the first half, I suspect that she knew she was late but deliberately jumped in order to intimidate. Certainly, there was no sign of remorse or an apology, neither while the blood was streaming out of my nose on the pitch nor after the game. Would I even recognise her if I saw her again? It has been more than nine months, but only now can I write about her actions without bitterness and rage.

That progress shows that one day I'll be able to think about the subsequent actions, or lack there-of, of my City United teammates without this pain and anger. My recovery has been two-fold: my brain repairing the physical damage cause by the incident and the emotional & psychological damage caused by the reaction of others. In hind-sight, I've struggled with the inept advice from the initial A&E to 'take a week off football', with the betrayal of trust & help by people I had considered close friends, and, finally, with my own reaction. My desire to 'get back to normal' quickly, while understandable, has probably contributed to this long recovery. The refusal to accept that I now have a brain injury to manage has been a difficult struggle.

It's been a year of facing hard truths, of adjusting to a new reality. I've lost friends, my sport, numerous career opportunities, and my phone. I've missed important events like births & weddings. But most of all I've lost my own sense of self. My personal 'invulnerability cloak' has taken a huge knock. I have a loving husband, a safe house, caring friends and a job waiting for me. My father would introduce me as someone for whom the glass is always half full. Yet I have still felt suicidal at some points. It has been that hard.

Equally I've done things I didn't expect. The bits I remember of the family holiday in Italy were wonderful. I've joined & enjoyed tai chi and, more startlingly, noticed a change in my posture and mind-set as a result. I didn't think I was someone who would attend meditation lessons at a Buddhist centre but, well, there we go.

Counselling was another first for 2014. Never thought I'd need it and certainly didn't think it would help so much. I don't enjoy the process but, wow, the results! Sometimes it's not till you say something out loud that you realise how silly it is – or how much of a hold it has over you. The improvement in my happiness levels since I had my first session in November! The regrets of not getting on to counselling or neurology referrals in those first six months after the incident may never go away. But, as Ash keeps reminding me, you can only go on what the medical professionals tell you at the time. Still the fight to get seen by a neurologist?! Nine weeks for the NHS to realise their booking system has me booked into a clinic that doesn't exist! Ah well, better not jinx it as haven't seen them yet.

The personal landmarks of recovery have been interesting. The first time I was able to listen to a song again; my first run in months – even if it was an unsuccessful sprint after the phone thief. These stick in my head. Keeping the diary has really borne fruit in that respect. Over the last few weeks, I've been looking back through it occasionally. The record of days passing does show the progress made, even if I missed it at the time. The diary has proven to be a great help as I've felt new slumps coming on. When I start to slide down again, I can look back and tell myself 'see you will come out of it, you are getting better'. It's also interesting to see how a slump now is like a good day three or four months ago. The energy gone in to writing up a diary each evening has been worth it and I'm glad I have a new one to start tomorrow.

I can feel I'm pushing it now. Dizziness again and I just caught myself gritting my teeth. Time to pop this diary away and start anew in the new year.

Resolution: I must improve my spelling.

2015: Priorities

Chapter 6

Finding a diagnostic pathway
Enter the specialists

January: Ten months after the incident

Diary entry

MONDAY: First counselling session of the new year and I'm not sure why I was expecting a gentle or 'light' session. I mean, the whole point of therapy is to deal with things that aren't gentle.

I spent the first few minutes pretending to be upbeat. I was trying to hide from everyone, even my counsellor. My hands wouldn't play along though, and spent the time tearing at tissues. After letting me act to a standstill, Willow drew out of me a confession that I was depressed.

'Do you usually feel sad at this time of year?'

'I was happy last New Year. But since then it has been hideous. Everyone has moved on, friends have married or had kids or got promoted or left me behind and disappeared. And I'm just stuck here, with everything wrong, and no answers and...'

There were no more tissues to shred. The remains floated to the floor, landing wherever the air currents took them. Willow let the silence settle with them. *I am in pieces, thin and ragged, and see through, and left to lie where I fall.*

'And what if... What if I keep getting everything wrong? Is this rock bottom?' *Please let it be, I don't think I can handle falling much further.*

Willow earned her buck then. 'It is ok to feel awful. It doesn't mean you've failed or that you've hit rock bottom. You are trying to make sense of a year which hasn't made sense in many ways. But you have done the best you could with what you had. Perhaps you could stop beating yourself up about it.'

'I don't know how to get out of here.'

'Sometimes we don't have all the information before making a decision but that doesn't make it wrong. We do know one thing. We know that 2015 will be a very different year for you.'

'I… hadn't thought of that.'

'How does it make you feel?'

'Scared. And excited.'

Patient's notes for first neurology appointment

- Have been effectively off work for 10 months and still having symptoms.
- Headaches daily and tinnitus fairly constantly but of varying strength.
- Fuzzy, unstable days several times a week.
- Funny spots in vision and seeing and hearing things.
- Not able to work, even from home due to dizzy and nausea spells.
- Social activity once a fortnight if that but need plenty of recovery time.
- Having good spells of maybe a week or so, followed by bad spells.

Diary entry

THURSDAY: Today was my first neurology appointment – at last! A long day and I feel drained, physically & emotionally. I had pinned so many hopes onto this appointment that I was awake most of the night. I suppose it was only natural to be nervous. Mum and Dad had given me a good pep talk and urged me to take someone else along. Someone else to listen in and remember things for me. With the husband working to pay the bills, I needed a friend. I'd met Peony a few years before and she had been sure to text and call regularly over the last year. Now she stepped up again and met me in the waiting room.

I found it difficult to keep a lid on my anxiety while we waited, but once my name was called the nurse was lovely and took a full hour to do a fairly thorough assessment. I found my anxiety didn't help me to stay calm during the appointment. I tried to stay focused and not let fear take over but it was difficult when talking about how bad things are. Turns out that the scan I went for in October was with a different NHS Trust. While a transfer of records had been requested, they had not yet been received. That was disheartening but the nurse said they would book me in for another one to check for changes anyway.

Immediate takeaways were that I should use less paracetamol & ibuprofen when self-medicating for headaches, as I was in danger of getting medication-overuse headaches. Murphy's law! But otherwise I should keep doing more of the same as I seem to be doing the right things. I could maybe add more structure to my days by napping at the same times for the same length. The nurse is putting in referrals for me to four different clinics. The letters for these will come through in the post.

The main change since the appointment is the relief. I've not been doing everything wrong, or making things worse or missed any huge problems. I'd also asked about the 'six-month window'. The response was that, while they would have preferred to see me sooner, there was no reason why the therapies would not have an effect, even a year on. I slept deeply during my afternoon nap and actually felt rested, the first time I've felt rested in a year. The on–off again question of work has been decided too. The nurse couldn't order me off, but made it plain that she felt I shouldn't return yet as I need a longer recovery. So, I'll need to call Alder to confirm and to sort the GP sick notes, but that can wait for now. I'm exhausted and am gritting my teeth to push through pain again. But tomorrow is a whole new day.

Clinic notes: Adult brain injury

Cognitively, the patient reports significantly reduced concentration and short-term memory problems. Emotionally she feels depressed and reports anxiety. Though this has improved with some external counselling support. She reports feeling very frustrated with the situation. We will refer her to the following clinics and review the situation in three months.
- Neuro-otology for dizziness treatments
- MRI brain injury sequence
- Neuropsychologist assessment
- Vocational rehabilitation

Diary entries

MONDAY: GP appointment today and was signed off for another three months. I know it is the best move but am still struggling with how long this is taking. That means that I definitely won't be back to a normal career for at least a year after the incident. Trying not to focus on that but it feels like a hell of a long unplanned career break.

This evening was the last of my six counselling sessions but Willow has asked me to take a further six. Given how in demand they are that was an indication of how much she thinks I need it. By the end of the session I'd decided she was right. I'm working on breaking the habits of thought and behaviour which I've developed as coping mechanisms and that is not easy. Willow also noted that I tend to apologise for being exhausted and dizzy during our sessions. It seems that stress is a trigger but she asked me to stop blaming myself for this happening. Homework this week is to relax and enjoy things without having to justify the enjoyment. Can I take this opportunity to change my habits and create a happy new life? Working on it!

TUESDAY: Had a long conversation with a friend today who is not happy and I don't know how to help. It seemed like she is very much where I was when I started counselling, that feeling that everything is a problem and there is always pressure to do something. It made me realise how much counselling has helped as I can see that pattern in others as well as myself now. And now that I can spot it, can I break the thought habit? Because that's what it is, a habit. Always reacting to pressure and expectation in an anxious 'I have to do everything, no-one's helping and the world is against me' way. I'll probably always need to catch myself and stop from reacting like that. But the rewards if I can do it! Very tired tonight with headache and tinnitus but am happier and accept them at the moment.

Email to parents

ME: Over here things are finally happening. It took ten months to get a neurological assessment, but in the week since, I've already had two referral appointments confirmed. Plus, I've received notification that I'm on the waiting list for a second MRI as the first scan is still missing. So good news that things are progressing.

I was feeling chipper about the progress, so treated myself to a garden centre visit; I deserved a nice outing. *Oh man, I'm 34 and using phrases like 'nice outing'. This injury is making me old.* Being out in public was strange after so long alone. I no longer felt comfortable and struggled to judge my behaviour. I analysed the bus driver's automatic grunt for clues. Was my cheery greeting appropriate? That passenger shifted seats when I got on, and the other woman has crossed her arms. Is that normal body language, or can they tell that there is something wrong with me? *Stop worrying!*

I couldn't. I was trying to soak up every nuance in the cramped space and my poor brain quickly went numb. At the next stop, I stumbled off the bus and managed to walk to the quiet park. Mercifully the nearest bench was empty, I sat with eyes closed while the panic slowly ebbed. Eventually, I was able to resume the slow journey.

Pottering round the garden centre brought an epiphany. *I'm afraid of accepting how things are in case I stop striving for how I want them to be.* I must accept that I can't do all that I want at the moment. I know where I would like to be and what I would like to do. Often, I am still questioning if I will ever be back to that normality. With all the change in the last year, that fear was to be expected. But worrying about the future prevents me from getting better now.

February: Eleven months after the incident

Diary entries

SUNDAY: A nice sleep in yesterday but reading for a few hours turned out to be a bad mistake. I had pushed my brain by asking it to read constantly and hadn't taken enough cognitive rest. The result was a surge of dizziness and exhaustion which left me scared and frustrated. So, I snapped at Ash and the day just got worse. This meant I spent Sunday trying to be more careful about how long I read and concentrate for. Turned once again to the timers as a way of ensuring breaks. During those rests I noticed that I have been brooding on the rejection from my old team a bit more. It is a habit I get into when I'm tired & depressed, like my defences are low and habitual thinking returns. But once I've noticed, I can sometimes pull myself out of it. Not a great few days but trying not to beat myself up. Very tired, lightheaded and disappointed in myself.

FRIDAY: Am feeling very lost and alone at the moment. The news that a colleague is having two scans within days of going private on his wife's work insurance has struck me like a blow. Glad he is getting the treatment but it makes me feel more stupid in the eyes of everyone at work and all those who urged me to go private. But it was much easier said than done with no insurance and the attempts I made at registering as a private paying customer were dealt with terribly. But don't I just feel like such a fool! I don't want to be spending my days alone and struggling, feeling caught in a trap. Trapped in the choices I did make and tormented by the possibilities of those I didn't. I have been invoking a bit more 'fantasy company' these last few days so must keep an eye on that – perhaps feeling a bit lonely again. The tinnitus and dizziness are here, my constant companions. I feel stretched and nauseous, not felt like that for a while.

Saturdays and Sundays were no longer filled with pubs, friends and football matches. The only difference on weekends was that Ash kept me company through the quiet hours of reading and gardening, interspersed with naps.

My news feeds and bookmarked websites had changed over the past year. I no longer checked up on football league tables and would search for research on brain injuries and treatments instead. Often it was a fruitless or confusing task as most articles were about brand-new treatments under development or incredible survivor stories. I hadn't been snatched from the jaws of death and needed help now, so most of the research, while heartening, was irrelevant.

That weekend I came across a reassuring and inspiring tale. A stroke survivor who had received an experimental therapy twenty years after their injury was suddenly able to dream again. A change in therapy, even so long after the initial stroke, had meant the brain could still heal, could now dream. News of such a dramatic improvement, so many years after the injury, was another reassurance that my treatment wasn't coming too late. Six months hadn't been the end of this patient's recovery and needn't be the end of mine. *I can still get better!* It was time to pick myself up and soldier on, again.

Diary entries

MONDAY: Counselling was interesting tonight. I still had the headache that had hung around through the day and felt a little dazed at the start of the session. However, I've noticed that strolling to counselling and sitting on the bus afterwards has become a time when all I have to do is think 'How am I?' Willow and I spoke about getting trust back in myself and in my relationships with others, which is definitely something that has seen progress. Also, I'm happier and have more time for the people who matter to me. Willow pointed out that I have no responsibilities to anyone but myself right now, which is very unusual for an adult. I feel an accompanying pressure to do something big and amazing. Everyone does that after a life changing injury, right? But really, the changes are for me and if I can feel well and be happy then that's great. Willow has also been giving me more homework now. She is asking me to write about how I feel and how I have power over my emotions. Our counselling sessions will come to an end so she wants me to get into the habit of doing this 'me time' on my own. Tired, tinnitus and dizzy again.

THURSDAY: Well, second day in a row where my head felt better than the last one. I took a quiet day on the sofa but that only aggravated my back pain. My sedentary lifestyle has led to a stiff and sore spine over the last few months. I have been itching to stretch it out and move a bit more, but need to find a way of doing that which felt safe and gentle. I've spent years walking past a yoga class at the local community centre and, this evening, I bit the bullet and joined in. I knew absolutely nothing about yoga but the teacher was welcoming and I enjoyed it. It feels great to be moving and working parts of the body again and I felt safe while working out. There is a beginners' workshop starting this weekend so I have signed up already. Pleased I went and in a rare good mood now, if exhausted.

The next day, the pleasure of waking up without back pain was tempered by a headache. It was a much slower day than I'd had for a long time. I was learning that, anytime you try something new after a brain injury, fatigue doubles down. All that learning is twice as tiring.

Sleep didn't seem to help as it was filled with disturbing and confusing dreams. As I said to Alder once, your brain does weird things when it is unwell. When I had stretched myself too far, my mood would sink and the anxiety was reflected in strange, sometime fearful, dreams. Those dreams would be hard to wake up from, as if the nightmares clung to the waking world.

But, on days when I had managed to rest enough, sleep was pleasant. A gift to look forward to. It was odd, this need to be rested in order to sleep well, but it was true. On good days my memories were coming back.

Each nap was a window in time. Memories long forgotten would reappear in my dreams. Places and people reminding me of who I was. Playing in the treehouse at the bottom of my childhood garden, enjoying the warm rays of a frosty sunrise after nightshift, working in a bustling wine store on a blazing hot afternoon. I began to look forward to sleep again.

Or memories might be triggered by a sound. I was able to listen to music now, but found that lyrics left me dazed. I couldn't work out what was being said so the speech washed over me. My playlists were all classical, as I searched for songs without lyrics. One day, the track flipped to Nyman's 'The Heart Asks Pleasure First'. I recognised it from the soundtrack to Jane Campion's 'The Piano.' Though I was in a tiny London flat, the song transported me back to a former home, a sprawling farm homestead on a hill station in New Zealand. We sat, my flatmates and I, rapt as a visiting Frenchman coaxed a pounding rhythm from the piano. That memory from half a world and half a lifetime away was another jigsaw piece, adding to the puzzle of who I was.

At the end of the month, Willow noticed this change too. She could see glimpses of a personality emerging from the fog of anxiety and fatigue.

'You smiled there. A real one, not a wry regret.'

'It felt right. It hasn't felt right to smile for a while now.'

'Why did it feel right now?'

'I dunno.'

She shifted; I knew that wasn't good enough. Willow needed a better answer, I deserved a better answer.

'I realise that I agonise over making decisions and face everything as if it is an "end of the world if you get it wrong" scenario. But it doesn't have to be that way. I know now that decisions can be changed and I can be happy with things just as they are. Things aren't perfect where I am now but they're getting better.'

'So you smiled because…'

'Because there is a way out.'

Chapter 7

Hospital appointments

You wait ages, then five come along at once

March: One year after the incident

Diary entry

MONDAY: A year to the day exactly since a striker squished my brain so I treated myself to a haircut. Seems like a silly thing to mark the occasion but I was trying to 're-boot' myself and get my life back. I also met Alder to discuss the possibility of returning to work next month. I'm not sure I want to go back to the same management role as it was very stressful. We'll see. I don't have to worry until April. Alder has been, and I'm sure will be, incredibly supportive. But his response is guided by me and I have no idea what the right answer is.

Last counselling session

'Where do you see yourself in a year's time. Where are you in March 2016?'

'2016?! I'm struggling with the fact that it is 2015. I feel like I've missed a year.'

'So much has happened, just not what you expected.' Willow stayed quiet while I thought that through. Her silence didn't scare me now, I'd grown comfortable with it. In the end, she was the one to speak. 'How have you been today?'

'I've been sad. This is our last session and you have been an important person in what has been a difficult time.'

'I feel privileged to have been a part of that time. To have been able to help you.'

'You, these sessions, have helped me so much. Thank you.'

'Do you feel you need more time, more sessions together?'

'Over the past few months, I've stopped looking backwards. 2016 is still too far away for me to think about. But I'm able to focus more on the present and the immediate future. The fact that I'm not stuck in that cycle of lament, well, I don't feel I need more sessions.'

'We are always here if you need, even an emergency session. But I agree. I think you are ready.'

'I feel ready to tackle what comes next, even though we don't know what that is. You got me there.'

'You did the hard work. All that is in this room is what you brought with you.'

That was true, looking back Willow kept herself out of the room. She learnt a great deal about me and helped me in ways I still don't understand. But I knew nothing about her. Where she lived, what she enjoyed doing. Initially I was terrified of running into her in a pub one day, this person who knows the darkest parts of me. But later I wanted to see her, to thank her. To show Willow the person we had sculpted during those long dark evenings.

At the same time as the counselling sessions finished, hospital appointments began to fill my calendar. After a year in the doldrums, I was in the NHS system and things started to happen at lightening pace. In the first week of March, I had my first appointment with a specialist brain injury clinic. I had a second appointment with them the next week and they discharged me.

This speedy turnaround was with the neuropsychologist team. At the first appointment I was given a series of written and oral tests over the course of two hours. It was exhausting, but resulted in good news.

At the follow up appointment, the neuropsychologist reported that I didn't present with any cognitive impairments. *Yay, my brain isn't too badly damaged!* Her suspicion was that the physical symptoms of dizziness and fatigue were breaking my concentration and preventing me from making new, or complete, memories. As she pointed out, if the brain is interrupted when it is making the memory then, even if the memory storage and recall is perfect, the memory will never be complete.

So, we were back to 'manage the symptoms' again. But that was making sense now. The neuropsychologist introduced me to the term 'cognitive lapse' and to the concept of 'false attributions'. A cognitive lapse happens to anyone. It is a fancy term for that moment when you walk into a room and forget what you went in there for. I'd been experiencing cognitive lapses in mid-sentence, forgetting the rest of the words that had been neatly lined up just a second ago.

I was told that people with a head injury like mine tend to have the same number of cognitive lapses as healthy people, but we blame them on our injury. We falsely attribute a fairly normal lapse to the fact that our brain is temporarily impaired. We blame ourselves, whereas someone with a healthy brain might laugh it off.

This blame can lead to more worry and anxiety, which can then interrupt the concentration. So, we have another lapse. Which leads to another false attribution and on it goes. This was another 'ah ha!' moment. *It's not that I'm forgetting something, everyone does that. It's that I'm beating myself up about my forgetfulness rather than paying attention to the next thing.*

I left the appointment determined to stop treating my cognitive lapses as a failure. It wasn't fool-proof, it didn't always work. But eventually I got into the habit of mental reassurance rather than blame. I still forgot things, but I was less anxious when I did and would no longer have a string of lapses in a row.

Diary entry

FRIDAY: A long day and today's appointment makes clinic number three, I think? I've seen adult ABI & neuropsychologist. Today was vocational rehabilitation with neuro-otology still to come. The appointment was exhausting as it took nearly an hour & a half and involved a lot of listening and comprehension. It is hard work, I hope to see some benefits soon!

Clinic notes: Vocational rehabilitation

The patient has developed avoidance behaviour of crowds and loud or busy environments. She has some difficulty negotiating escalators & stairs and social activities have been limited by fatigue. The patient has been off work for over a year but is keen and motivated to return. When discussing her failed return attempts, it was found that, while she was at reduced hours, the complexity & volume of duties were not similarly reduced. The patient found that the stress of the job was a trigger for her symptoms which led to cycle of vestibular symptoms, fatigue and associated anxiety. I have suggested that the patient remain off work for now. We will commence work-hardening tasks such as completing computer work and writing to test her concentration in anticipation of returning to work.

The four 'P's' of fatigue management

Sometimes, those parts of a medical consultation which are valued most by the patient are never mentioned in the records. The clinic notes don't reveal that both the neuropsychologist and the vocational rehabilitation therapist spent over two hours with me. It isn't recorded that they listened and explained and reassured and sent me home with a plan to manage my fatigue.

Firstly, I was told that it was important to sustain a moderate level of activity to avoid a 'boom and bust' cycle of fatigue. I found it helpful to think of fatigue management as managing your percentage of effort. Gym classes and personal trainers sometimes do this in a class e.g. 'we'll do 50% in a warm up and then go all out, 100%, in the middle.'

When managing fatigue, it is better to potter along at a steady 60 or 70% of effort than to cycle between 100% and 30%. This means not having a huge spike of activity when you are feeling good. Instead, think of it as 'banking your energy' for later.

This helps with recovery as well. The vocational rehabilitation team used another metaphor for recovery, the phone battery. You might have noticed that a phone will take proportionally longer to recharge when the battery is nearly dead. A recharge from 50% might take an hour, but a recharge from 10% might take ten times as long. It is the same when recovering from fatigue. As we use more energy up, each hour takes longer to recover from than the last.

Also, it can help take small, frequent breaks rather than pushing through several hours and then collapsing for a long time. I was advised to take a break every 20–30 minutes rather than hourly. Makes sense, but the bit that always tripped me up, was that it should be a cognitive break, 'a rest for the brain too.' This meant having a proper break of doing nothing, not switching from one task to another, or from the computer to the phone.

Finally, the team told me about the importance of balancing out the activities. This meant balancing them throughout the day and the week to help you avoid a 'boom and bust.' But the balancing also refers to fun. There are always tasks which need to be done, even when recovering from a brain injury we need to make food or wash clothes. We need to do those things and also make sure we do other tasks that we enjoy too. This helps to ensure you get pleasure or a sense of accomplishment, that it isn't all just jobs and schedules. It took me a while to come around to the idea of 'planned fun'. In a brain injury recovery, it is indispensable.

Essentially, this advice boiled down into setting your Priorities, Planning out what needs to be done, and Pacing your time so you get to have fun and rest too. I was told these are 'the three 'P's' of fatigue management'. After a good think, I decided something was missing. To me it seemed to be the most important one. Because, how can you work out what your priorities are if you don't have any Perspective? You need to know what is most important to you before you can prioritise them in your day.

1. Perspective
2. Priorities
3. Planning
4. Pacing

It was daunting, where to start? Well, 'begin at the beginning,' as the King in Wonderland told Alice. I knew there would be plenty of naps before we got to the end.

Perspective can be a tricky thing. Are we viewing the world from the right angle? Has something happened which affects that outlook? The problem with a personal perspective is that it is personal. I can't tell you how to find perspective but sometimes we need help to get there. My time with Willow had helped me to work through the changes of the last year to realise that I just want to be happy again. Of course, we can't be happy all the time, that's impossible. But I knew that I'd like to hold onto things that made me happy.

So, what makes me happy? Willow and I had worked that out as well, though I don't think I'd ever written them down before. The first one was obvious, how many times had I said 'I just want to feel normal again.' So priority number one was my health.

Getting structure

The vocational rehabilitation team had given me a weekly Fatigue Management Planner which covered every hour of every day for a week and told me to plan out my time. Good health is laudable, but it isn't a meeting. How do you plan it out over a week?

Well, to be healthy we need to get enough sleep. This is particularly true during a recovery from brain injury. I had to be up a regular time and still needed at least nine hours of sleep a night. So, the hours of 10pm to 7am were blocked out. Good hygiene, exercise and food were all important and they took up more hours. I had hospital and doctor appointments to plug into the Planner, as well as the travel time needed.

Good health means good mental health too, and the vocational rehabilitation team had said the schedule needed to include things I find fun. I added in time for my hobbies: gardening, learning a new language, playing my cello and reading. By the time all of these were planned in, along with rest periods after each one, the days were nearly full. But I'd only managed to fit in one priority!

While staring at my list of hobbies, I realised that my mental health also improved when I spent time with Ash and my friends. So, priority one was trimmed back to bare essentials, exercise and hospital appointments. This gave me time for priorities two and three: Husband and Friends. As my recovery progressed and the frequency of hospital appointments dropped, I was able to spend more of my time on the people and hobbies that I love.

Diary entry

MONDAY: Another new clinic today. They are all in the same hospital and the entry staff know me by sight already. The letter requested that I be there for 8:45 and to expect a long morning. They even recommended bringing snacks.

I reported to the clinic and tried to pronounce the name 'neuro-otology.' The receptionist smiled, 'we just say dizzy docs' and guided me to the waiting room.

In between the waiting, there were lots of tests. Hearing tests, sight tests, being strapped into a chair and spun around in the dark tests. The worst was the 'caloric' test where water is squirted into the ears to deliberately induce dizziness. It was exactly like those awful months early on when the world just span constantly. Fortunately, it abated quickly while I sat in the waiting room, but I felt delicate for a few hours.

Once all the results were in, I was called in for the final verdict. Apparently, I tested very well on the ears and eyes. The only concern was that my visual tracking of an object is quite jumpy. They called it a 'mildly broken sight pursuit'. *There's that mild again! You try it, it isn't fun!*

The doctor then spoke about 'vestibular migraine'. I had trouble following what caused it. From what I could make out, the dizziness gives you a migraine and then the migraine makes you dizzy, which gives you a migraine… Treatment is about breaking that cycle. *I have so many cycles to break.*

I might not understand vestibular migraines fully, but I am so relieved to have a name for this. *It has a name. This thing I have. Which actually exists! And there might be a solution!* The neuro-olotogist spoke about 'migraine prophylactics', pills to help prevent migraines which he thought would really help.

I didn't escape the hospital until mid-afternoon as, once the dizzy doc team were done, the radiology team said they could fit me in. So, I finished the day with another 30mins spent in a magnet, hopeful that this MRI wouldn't also go missing.

Clinic notes: Neuro-otology/dizzy docs

Clinical findings:

• Episodic headache.
• Vertigo.
• Soft central vestibular signs.
• Mildly broken sight pursuit.
• Mildly impaired vestibular-ocular-reflex suppression.

Plan and recommendations

• MRI requested.
• I would recommend migraine prophylaxis; either Amitriptyline or Pizotofen.
• Referral for vestibular physiotherapy and cognitive behavioural therapy. I would like the vestibular physiotherapy team to include gaze stabilisation exercises to reduce the vestibular/visual conflict.
• Patient should keep a migraine diary of headaches and dizziness.

Migraine diary

I'd told the doctors that I was already keeping a diary of what happened day to day. But that wasn't what they meant. A migraine diary isn't a diary of appointments nor is it a place for your daily thoughts and feelings. While a migraine diary does record headaches and dizziness, the real purpose to record where you are, what you are doing and what you have eaten when you feel dizziness or a headache start up. You do all this in the hope that you can start to identify what triggers your headaches and migraines. It sounded exhausting, especially when I felt I was barely able to make it out of bed on some days.

'So, I've got more homework? Can't you just give me the pills?'

'We are sorting out pills, but they can only partially work. To give yourself the best chance of reducing migraines, you need to work out what triggers them too.'

Priority one: do what I need to do to be in good health.

'Ugh, right. More homework.'

'Fortunately there is an app for that.'

Actually, there were hundreds. A quick search of the web and app stores turned up a bewildering array of results. I decided to use a market leader, and it proved to be thorough and easy to use. I was very happy with it. Until an update added in a chat forum. Initially I was bombarded with notifications. Every time someone posted a comment I was notified. I managed to turn off notifications but the app was still downloading them in the background. It burnt through a month's worth of phone data in less than a week.

I decided to build my own migraine diary and it proved to be quite easy. I started with a simple spreadsheet. Days at the top and triggers down the side. The neuro-otology team had handily given me a list of the most common triggers and, as I read more on the NHS website, I added new ones in.

If I got a migraine that day, I would simply mark in the possible triggers I'd been exposed to beforehand. By the end of the month the sheet showed that I got about two migraines a week, which lasted for about 36 hours. Most of my migraines started when I was out in public or stressed, and I would see odd sparkles in my eyes just before they hit. My main triggers were: not enough sleep, being in busy or brightly lit places, cold temperatures, and, as for many women, my menstrual cycle.

Though I had initially resented the need for more homework, seeing some solid data on a page was a revelation. The sparkles in my vision were a sign that a migraine was coming on. Now when I saw them, I knew I should head home, or go back inside and have a nap. If I could manage that, then the migraines would usually be shorter. I also started to wear more clothes. Where I used to be comfortable in a t-shirt and jumper, I'd add in another layer. If that extra bit of warmth would help me to avoid migraines it was worth it. It was simple, and it worked. I wouldn't have known to try it if I hadn't done my homework.

My overriding emotion was relief at seeing real numbers on a page. This data showed the world that my migraines and symptoms were actually happening. It wasn't all in my head.

Reference

Carroll, L. (1865). *Alice's Adventures in Wonderland*. London: Macmillan

Chapter 8

Dizziness and related treatments

It's all in your head

Knowledge is a super power. I'd just been calmed and reassured by evidence that my attacks of headache and dizziness were both tangible and trackable. As I discovered more about my brain injury and related symptoms, I felt I had more control and my anxiety dropped.

This curiosity and need for more information took me to a presentation about dizziness hosted by a local brain injury group. The speaker was Dr. Barry Seemungal, neurologist at Imperial College London, who provided both information and encouragement. I was enthused by what I learned.

Summary of Dr. Seemungal's presentation on imbalance and dizziness after brain injury

Dizziness, is it all in my head? Actually, yes!

While many people associate dizziness and balance problems with the inner ear, or the vestibular organ, this is only part of the story. It is the brain which processes the information from your inner ear, limbs and eyes to maintain your balance. If the signals from the ears, eyes or limbs, or the brain mechanisms that process this information, are disturbed we may feel dizzy or off balance or even both.

So, dizziness and imbalance are not the same thing?

For the purposes of clarity, we can define dizziness as 'the illusion of moving when you are not'. So, dizziness is a sensation or a feeling that you are moving when in fact you are standing still. An example of motion might be feeling like you are on a merry go round or a rocking boat.

This defined use of the word dizziness contrasts with its everyday usage which can mean light headedness or intelligence – e.g. 'a dizzy blonde'.

It is important that the doctor understands that dizziness can understood in different contexts by the public and patients.

Imbalance is the inability to maintain a stable posture when standing still or walking, sometimes with the risk of falling. Balance is a complex and difficult task, taking human babies over a year to learn, and much longer to master. It is therefore not surprising that any disturbance to brain functioning often leads to imbalance and falls.

Feeling imbalanced does not always mean that we are imbalanced

A feeling of being imbalanced usually means that the brain is correctly telling us that we are at risk of falling. Perhaps because the body is tilted too much and we need to make a small correction with our legs to maintain our stability. But sometimes, even if the motor system provides accurate information to our muscles and there is no real risk of falling, the brain's monitoring system will wrongly think we are imbalanced. It will tell us we are at risk of falling when we are not. Or the opposite may happen, where a person has impaired balance but is not aware of it and hence may be at risk of falling and injury.

Further, balance is visible to all whereas dizziness is a very personal thing and is only felt by the patient. Sometimes dizziness will be associated with imbalance, but sometimes you can feel dizzy with normal balance. This means that you can be standing steadily, and a doctor may assess your balance as being normal, but you feel dizzy.

The brain is the organ of balance

A feeling of instability is a common and often debilitating symptom of brain injury. Walking is a risky business, even for a healthy person who isn't experiencing dizziness or imbalance. Every time we step, we nearly fall. To walk, our brain's motor system must send signals to our muscles to contract and move the limbs. At the same time, there is a system in the brain that monitors our balance in response to our movements.

Once we know our brain is the organ of balance, we can start to understand how it works. Our brain interprets what we see and feel in a logical way. It evolved this way over millions of years. So really, we have:

A caveman's brain in the modern world

Take the example of our distant ancestor running away from a tiger in the jungle. Their eyes will see lots of trees flying past at high speed. The brain needs to work out that the trees can't move so it must be the person who is moving. Feedback from the running limbs helps the brain to work out it is the person moving and not the trees. This sense of our limb position is the most important sense for our balance. Other senses can help too; the feel of the air rushing past and the growls of the tiger, hopefully, fading into the distance.

In the modern world the brain can sometimes find it hard to work out whether it is the person or environment that is moving. Take the situation of a person standing on a platform and watching a train race past. The speeding train fills most of the vision and the brain needs to distinguish whether the person or the train is moving. On occasions, this proves difficult and the brain comes up with the wrong answer. It thinks the train can't be moving, so the person must be. Thus, the brain creates the illusion of self-movement and the person feels dizzy.

Chronic dizziness and imbalance

Dizzy patients who do not receive the right treatment can adopt compensatory strategies which are not always useful. For example, it is common to rely more on our vision for our balance after an episode of dizziness. This can, over time, make us overly sensitive to environments which have lots of visual stimuli. Examples of such an environment might be supermarket aisle full of different products, crowded places or shopping malls. This makes it even more important to access the right treatment.

Treat the things you can treat!

Dizziness is not something you have to put up with. In fact, many causes of dizziness can be treated and cured. Depending on the type of dizziness, treatment options may include vestibular physiotherapy and/or medications. Patients struggling with vestibular physiotherapy should note that it does work, even if it doesn't feel like it at first. Often the exercises are designed to make you feel dizzy, which can be unpleasant and scary and can feel as if you are getting worse not better.

It is important to get the order treatment correct as sometimes a person with poorly controlled migraines may find that the vestibular physiotherapy triggers migraines and makes their dizziness worse. In such cases, it may be helpful to control the migraines with medication before embarking on a course of vestibular rehabilitation.

To make sense of this, it might help to think of your vestibular system as being similar to your immune system. As you are gradually exposed to a cold or virus, you feel awful. However, over time your body becomes better at fighting the virus and you start to get better. You might even be able to resist catching that bug in future. So too with the vestibular system and dizziness. Your body becomes better at fighting the dizziness and over time your balance improves, making you feel less dizzy. This process can take weeks or more likely months, rather than days.

Studies on ballet dancers show that the balance area of the brain changes as they train. This is known as brain plasticity, when the brain can change in response to training. For the brain to change in this way, you need to do a lot of training so any dizziness or balance exercises you do should be fun. Taking physical exercise and getting enough sleep are also useful to keep your balance senses trained.

Dizziness, imbalance and mental health

Experiencing dizziness or imbalance can be terrifying, not just because of the symptoms, but because the centres controlling our emotions have links to areas which process dizziness and imbalance.

Let's go back to our ancestor running from the tiger in the jungle. If the ancestor has trouble with balance or feels dizzy, they will have much less chance of escaping the tiger. Evolution has bred us to panic or become anxious when we can't run or walk, or if we have balance problems.

For this reason, balance problems are often interlinked with anxiety and depression. This link is important as in some cases the anxiety and depression must be treated at the same time as the dizziness to have the best possible recovery.

Dizziness, imbalance and fatigue

Dizziness and imbalance can amplify problems with pathological fatigue following an ABI. Normal fatigue is not chronic and sleep or rest will alleviate it. Pathological fatigue is common after a brain injury and can be present most of the time. While rest will help, it will not remove pathological fatigue.

This pathological fatigue presents in different ways, and to differing levels, following an ABI. In those people who also have a dizziness or imbalance problem, the fatigue is often worse. This is perhaps because the brain reserve is used up with trying to deal with the imbalance and dizziness.

In conclusion:

- The link between brain injuries and dizziness or imbalance is clear.
- You don't have to live with dizziness! It can be treated, but first your doctor should provide a precise list of the causes (or diagnoses) for your dizziness.

- Dizziness is not a non-specific symptom of head injury; it has specific diagnoses and specific treatments.
- As your treatment progresses and you improve, you may develop new symptoms that were previously hidden by the dizziness and imbalance. Or you may start feeling worse because, now that you are able to do more, you end up doing too much. This irregular progression to recovery is quite normal. Your therapist can help you navigate your way through this irregular path to recovery.

Doctor Seemungal's talk was enlightening. Finally, there was an explanation as to why I was dizzy after seeing certain triggers. And he showed me that I would be able to treat my symptoms.

Clinic notes: Vestibular physiotherapy

The patient has been referred for vestibular physiotherapy having sustained a football head injury in March 2014. Approximately two days following the injury she experienced acute severe persistent vertigo with the sensation of tilt and feeling her eyes were sliding to the left. Since the initial onset of symptoms seventeen months ago they have resolved significantly.

Today the patient was educated on the balance systems and postural control in relation to the assessment finding. We discussed the principles of vestibular physiotherapy and hope that with approximately three more follow ups we will be able to get her back to a very high level of baseline balance function. She was provided with a simple home exercise programme to get started with before we see her again.

It is a cliché to save the best till last, but that is what happened with my hospital appointments. I had seen the other clinics multiple times before an initial assessment with the vestibular physiotherapy team could be scheduled.

The vocational rehabilitation therapist had repeatedly said that vestibular physiotherapy would make a marked difference to my symptoms. She had also noted how well I was doing for someone who hadn't had any as yet. So, it was with high spirits that I embarked on their instructions.

The physiotherapist urged me to try getting out a bit more and that I would keep improving by adding in new things to test my limits. She told me that I need to remember the bubble of support and avoidance behaviour which builds up around someone with a brain injury can still be a cage.

Obviously, I couldn't pick up all my tasks at once. As with everything else, I needed a plan. The physio helped with a few rules:

- Try one new thing every week and give it a week to bed in.
- Build up slowly (e.g. if you want to return to cycling, try doing an extra kilometre a week).
- Learn to love 'planned spontaneity'. Meaning plan in days with activities, days without activities where I can do what I feel like and days for resting in between.
- Schedule in the social stuff over a month ahead so you have time to plan for it and think about it.

Vestibular exercises

As well as notes on organising my diary, I now had new exercises to fit in every day. These exercises were designed to improve my gaze stabilisation as well as my static and dynamic balance. Static balance helps us to remain still when standing or sitting, while dynamic balance keeps us steady while moving around. There were standing and walking exercises, exercises with spinning umbrellas and exercises where I watched videos of other people moving.

I said that this was both the last and best clinic. It was the best because these exercises alleviated my dizziness more than any other treatment. This relief then helped my fatigue, which in turn helped everything else. But it was also the worst clinic.

As Dr Seemungal's talk had explained, the way to treat dizziness is by making someone dizzy and training the senses to resist the sensation. The aim of these exercises was to push me into being dizzy, but not too dizzy. If I was dizzy for longer than 20 minutes, or if I got a headache, then I was doing too much and should reduce the difficulty of the exercise. But the only way to know if the exercises were too much was to do them. Three times a day, every day.

After the first couple of tries, I found a level of exercise that fitted the 'dizzy, but not too dizzy' criteria. I also found that it takes half an hour to do the full set of exercises and then about another half an hour to recover. This meant booking in three hours across each day for them. The struggle to do these at a fairly regular time and still fit in all the hospital appointments meant rearranging the Fatigue Management Planner again. After months of loneliness and inactivity, my days were now filled with therapies and their side effects.

Vestibular migraines and the trippy pills

The neuro-otology/dizzy doc clinic had diagnosed me with vestibular migraine. To my layman's understanding, these migraines meant that I had basically lurched between migraines and dizziness, or both, for the last year. While it was a relief to finally have a 'thing with a name', even better was walking back from the pharmacist with my first box of migraine prophylactics, or migraine prevention pills.

Dr Seemungal noted that there are several drugs that can be used to prevent migraine, each with their own specific side effects that may suit a patient's differing needs. The dizzy docs agreed that amitriptyline was the drug most suited to my symptoms and I was relieved to be able to try them.

The box contained 28 tiny blue pills neatly arranged in blister packs. *Can pills so small really do anything?* The accompanying leaflet listed an impressive number of side effects. *That'd be a 'yes' then.* I admit to a wry chuckle when I read that the common side effects included headaches and dizziness. *Seriously?!* But the dizzy docs had emphasised that they believed these pills would help me. And I'd just spent a year hoping for a magic pill to make everything better.

All the sources of information I could find on amitriptyline, which included the dizzy docs, my GP, the medication leaflet, and lengthy online chat forums, emphasised that the pills made you sleepy. The GP went a little further:

'Drowsiness will be a big problem when you first start to take the pills. The key is to take the pills at a regular time in the evening. You'll find that after a few hours you will just want to sleep.'

She was right. After months of lying awake in bed the amitriptyline sent me to sleep easily. I slept long and deeply, but woke feeling groggy and numbed. My first week on these pills was another run of hazy drowsy days where I could barely feed myself in the morning. After a month or so, I had worked out that the drowsiness started about two hours after taking the pills and I was effectively out of action for about ten hours. As I wanted to be up and alert at 7.30am, I needed to set reminders to take the pills at 7.30pm. It worked, and after another week I was more lucid in the mornings. However, my brain switched off like a light at 9.30 in the evening. The Fatigue Management Planner needed re-working for the umpteenth time so I could fit everything in before then.

Once I had worked out how to manage the drowsiness, I noticed a few other side effects. The best was that any remaining hallucinations morphed into a kind of general happy 'high'. Instead of shadows moving in the corner of my eye, everything was now viewed with a technicolour filter. It was like the old 'Wizard of Oz' film when you suddenly swirl from dreary Kansas to a happy fantasy land. One day, I was on a bus in the late afternoon and the trees cut the low sunlight into vivid strips of dark and light. That strobing effect, and the surreal feeling from the pills, sent me into a happy trance and I missed my stop.

Another side effect was seriously trippy dreams. The 'wake covered in sweat and desperate for dawn to chase the nightmares away' kind of dreams. Those were far less fun and clung to my waking hours. The dreams seemed to be keeping me asleep as I struggled to wake and would finally do so with alarming suddenness. I was terrified during one nightmare that someone was in the house and I was fighting to get up and confront them but couldn't wake.

One morning I didn't recognise my face in the mirror. I mean, I knew it was me but something was definitely odd or missing. *Is that what people see when my brain blanks out? I know they see something cause they either worry or avoid me.* Every morning another new dream, leaving me horribly disturbed and questioning everything I saw or felt. *Am I pouring this cup of tea, or just dreaming that I am?*

It was horrible but I stuck with the pills for a very good reason, they seemed to be working. After a year of dizziness being problem number one, that spot was now taken by fatigue. I was still dizzy, but it was more manageable than the month before starting the amitriptyline.

As I emerged from the fog of dizziness and then drowsiness, I realised I was doing more than just coping. There were days when I felt happy again. I was more hopeful than I'd been since the incident, and was more fun to be around too. Life wasn't a constant struggle which was a huge difference compared to the last year.

And on the harder days, the bed ridden days, I was aware of the symptoms and would no longer just shoulder them and struggle on. Instead of somewhere I resented, bed became relief. A place to rest and get better. The tree outside was budding, just as it had been a year ago when the long, lonely hours in bed began. *Here I am again, but this time, with hope.*

Reference

Seemungal, B. (2017). *Imbalance and dizziness after brain injury.*

Chapter 9

Returning to former activities
Get out, do more stuff!

April: Thirteen months after the incident

Diary entry

WEDNESDAY: Just realised I've planned something in for the future! Something that is just for me and that I have no fears over. At our last session, Willow had asked me to start looking forward. I've now managed to do just that without a thought or an anxious 'should I?' moment. Great! Must admit I'm tired now. When I stop and close my eyes for a few seconds I can feel the tension in my teeth, mouth and back. I sense myself clamping down on the tinnitus and start of a headache. My usual way of coping so I can soldier on and get things done. Still a struggle to do things – definitely tired – bed time again. Rest day tomorrow.

Assault

The walls had been closing in again, that feeling of cooped up loneliness. The constant battle between the need to remain a part of this world and the fear of what might happen beyond the door. *Don't be silly*. I knew that I needed to move, to get some fresh air.

The supermarket was only a 10-minute walk away and I was having a dizzy-free spell. I walked slowly, feeling each step carefully. The shopping list was fairly long, we needed the weekly shop and an easter egg as a treat. While it took time, in the end it was fairly easy. The walk back home was slower, bags of food weighed me down. But I was happy, an unfamiliar feeling of late. As was my pride in myself. *You managed that, you handled it. Smiled at the cashier, just a normal person doing normal things.*

I imagined clinical notes that might be written up:

> Patient was able to plan meals for the week and buy the correct ingredients which showed evidence of cognitive function. She further demonstrated the ability to conduct herself in public and handle social situations without the other participants being aware of any impairment.

As I neared home, a plastic spoon flew out of a parked car in front of me. I picked it up and dropped it back through the window with 'hey, you dropped this.' I kept walking but heard a car door open behind me, the thump of feet landing on concrete.

'You b*tch!' came the shout.

Umm. Just keep walking normally.

'You f*cking b*tch!' The shouts were closer.

Despite my resolve, I increased my pace. Sweaty palms meant the shopping bag handles began to slip. *What the hell? And why did I buy so much?*

'I should f*cking hit you.' The footsteps sped up. 'Think you can get away, gonna f*cking whack you.'

*Sh*t, he's right behind me! What do I do? Turn round at least see the prick.*

He was tall and furious. At least seeing me turn stopped him. I was only a few steps out of his reach now.

'What the f*ck…?' I started

'You b*tch, f*cking throwing sh*t.'

'You threw a spoon out your car, I dropped it back in.'

'F*cking attacking people.'

'Me?! No, it's you. You leapt out of your car and chased me. You're the one shouting about attacking someone.'

'F*ck you, you piece of…' Spit was already flying from his mouth, and he gobbed a slimy mass of it towards me.

'Leave me alone, you crazy f*cker.'

'You know what, f*ck you.'

With that he lunged at me. I saw the fist coming, but hands full of shopping bags could do nothing to stop it. The backpack meant I couldn't sway away, and the impact shuddered through my face and nose.

Oh shit. Not there, not again. No, no, no, I was just getting better.

The world started spinning. I dropped the shopping and felt the warmth of blood stream out of my nose. The man had backed off but he was still close. Grinning horridly.

'See b*tch, f*cking told you.'

I ignored the metallic taste, the red drops on the pavement and managed to get my phone out. The video I took shows him threatening me with more punches. I'm shouting back at him and reading out the number plate of his car. He lunges forward. Two other men, bystanders who had been talking a few doors down, dart into shot. My attacker struggles against them as they form a barrier between the two of us. Eventually he gives up, gets into his car and races away.

The bystanders look at me, then walk away, back to their own world. As I retrieve my bags, I find an unfamiliar phone under the spilled groceries. The lock screen shows a photo of my attacker, smiling. I don't want to touch it. But it is more proof of who he is. In the end I pick it up with a bloodied tissue, I was onto my third by this point. *The police will know what to do with it. Police, yes, I need to call them.* But I wasn't safe here. *Once he realises the phone is missing, he'll come back!* I grip the bags with shaking hands and turn to the two bystanders. They stop talking as I approach.'Thank you for getting him away from me. I really appreciate that.' They nodded. 'Umm, I'm going to call the police, will you please speak to them?'

They weren't looking at me now. The pavement was more interesting than a woman with blood smeared across her face. The silence went on.

'Um, or can I take your details to give to them? Please? Just as witnesses... you know? ... Please.'

They glanced at each other, then back at the ground.

'Please. I've just been attacked.'

One turned and walked away quickly. *What?* ... The other had the balls to say 'No' before turning into his garden path.

'Please. He'll get away with it.'

The man kept walking.

'Please!'

He turned at last. 'Look we helped, but don't want to get involved.'

'Wh...Why?'

He shrugged. 'Didn't see much.'

'Didn't see much? You had to drag him off me!'

He looked at his shoes.

'We ain't talking to the police.' The door closed, a new trickle of blood ran into my open mouth.

I managed to get home, despite stopping often to check I wasn't followed. The constables arrived just before my anxious husband. Taking statements from a battered woman was depressingly routine for them but even so, a stranger 'attacking a woman on her own in broad daylight' was a new one on them. Another first with the police that I didn't need.

The man had punched me in exactly the same place as the injury which had started all of this a year previously. Once the police were finished, the fear of any further damage sent me back to hospital for yet more scans.

Diary entry

WEDNESDAY: Tired tonight, but not quite as wiped out as yesterday, and nowhere near as bad as the nights after the man hit me. Fortunately, the X-rays showed that my nose wasn't broken again. They didn't have room for me in the MRI, not a surprise at A&E on a Friday night. But I'm in the system for another MRI soon, so will find out about any more damage then. It is a worry, but I find it is my tiredness that gets me down at the moment. It is hard to be chipper when exhausted. I have been dizzier, and the headaches are worse. Seem to be unsteady on my feet too. Also, my teeth are hurting, I must be clenching them again. That isn't surprising as I'm definitely stressed with all the hospital visits finally happening. I also spend hours lying awake at night trying not to relive the assault. Feel lost again, there have been few moments of 'I must do something' or 'I should get out there!' But I seem to be better at noticing when I can do things and when I really just need to stop. Which is very encouraging! Last night I was struggling with a feeling of desolation, that I'm not having an impact on anything at the moment, that the world will just keep on going if I just stay in bed. But I've been fighting that feeling for months now and it is getting easier. Plus, I recognise it for what it is – a symptom of fatigue and not a fact. Getting there slowly and, despite the assault, I can tell that I'm getting back to myself so there is less fear in the question 'will I ever be myself again?'.

Email to Hazel

ME: Sorry for being a bit absent recently. Lots of doctor appointments in last few weeks. I'm not going back to work till at least end of May. That might be extended though as I've finally seen the vocational rehabilitation clinic. They have assigned me homework as part of a 'back to work plan'. The doctors want me to get 'work ready' by using the computer for extended work-like tasks – such as writing to friends!

So yes, lots of clinics now but also lots of waiting in receptions or for letters and phone calls. My goodness, I'm being forced to learn patience! Current wait is that I'm expecting to hear from another neuro team because an MRI taken before the assault showed a bruise in the brain. A worrying development to be sure, I'm hoping the prick punching me didn't make it worse. The registrars will meet to discuss it and are still trying to get hold of my scan from October. I'm trying to be calm but have to admit to a lot of fear. I still question if I did the right thing and feel guilt about any possible damage I might have caused after the injury. I'm haunted by the possibility of something having been missed on the first scan, which is still mysteriously absent.

I also received news that a new friend with a brain injury had settled out of court for the mistakes made in her treatment. So, I suppose it is natural for me to think along those lines too. After listening to me pour out these worries, Ash set me straight with 'wait until you know there has been a mis-diagnosis and then worry'. Very sensible, I just can't get to that reasoning by myself at the moment.

In good news, my nose is back to normal size and is still fairly straight. I seem to have a sense of smell so perhaps I won't need a career change. Plus, I don't need painkillers for the bruising any more. The black eyes have nearly gone so I no longer look like The Emperor from Star Wars. I've asked my GP to release all the records of my injury in the last year to the police. Figured if the scumbag who attacked me gets more time for hitting someone who is recovering from a head injury, then good!

The police have caught the bastard. He was easy to identify from the video and licence plate. Plus, they know him as he has a history of violence against woman and dishonesty offences. And he was out on bail when he attacked me. It took a while to find him though, he skipped his parole immediately after the assault and went into hiding. When the police tracked him down, he claimed that I attacked him and that any injuries he inflicted were in self-defence. Given his previous, and his skipping bail, he isn't believed. So, I haven't been charged with attacking a man taller and stronger than me while I was weighed down with shopping and long-term injury. But, as the witnesses refused to come forward, we have to go to court in early September – fun! For now, he is back in jail for his previous offence which has made me feel much better. I wish I was at work as it might be less stressful!

May: Fourteen months after the incident

Summary of emails with employer's HR team

HR: I'm completing the Statutory Sick Pay form for the end of your twenty-eight weeks of sick pay. Before I complete the form, I just want to make sure that we both agree the final date. I calculate 28 weeks to finish on the 14th June.

ME: Thank you for the email, and yes, I also calculate that the twenty-eight weeks finishes on the 14th of June. As an update, my doctor has renewed the sick note to the 1st of July and I will send a copy in the post. I am working through a plan for a return to work with the vocational rehabilitation team and will update you on any changes.

Diary entries

MONDAY: A bit of a funny day which started with a visit to the GP. She took my excitement and over-exuberance in her stride and helped bring me back down to earth to decide on a sensible course of action. At the recommendation of the vocational rehabilitation team I'm now off until July. I still find each milestone of not getting back to work a bit stressful, it feels like a failure despite all the obvious progress elsewhere. The sick note today was another blow. I found myself counting the months and regretting them. But it makes sense. The GP is on the case with trying to find my missing MRI scan from October and has also suggested a slight increase in the pills to try and stop the migraines and dizziness I'm still getting. Anyway, all this means I'd had a headache by the time I got home so big nap after lunch. Afternoons seem to be my best time as I managed to complete both sets of the vestibular physiotherapy exercises and the vocational rehabilitation homework. Pleased I managed it but now feeling really drained.

SUNDAY: Spent the weekend playing catch-up. After the GP recommended increasing the amitriptyline on Monday, this week has seen an increase in the vivid dreams to match. My mornings are just disappearing, lost in a haze of stupor and delirium. Saturday was awful. But the problem wasn't that I was exhausted and migraine-y. I mean, I was but I've dealt with that before and much worse so many times. The problem yesterday was that I didn't change my expectations to match my exhaustion. I was full of all the things I wanted to do or that I felt I had to get done. So, I wasn't letting myself slow down like I need and it just kept spiralling, till in the end I had to go to bed. Self-combustion.

Email to parents

ME: My visits to the respective doctors went well this week. The vocational rehabilitation therapist was pleased to hear that I would be off work until July – at last someone who was pleased with that news! She has also kept my 'getting ready for work' homework at two hours a day. It's not much but exhausts me every time. For someone who used to play full weekends of footy tournaments I still get annoyed at needing a nap after a reading a few emails or a taking a walk. But this slow road is definitely heading towards recovery and I am better than I used to be.

The appointment also made it clear that I've been pushing myself so it's nice not to feel like I have to keep doing so. The therapist also said I need to be a lot more stable in my breaks. Seems that while I can do cognitive rest well, I need to remember that my vestibular functions need rest too by lots of being still. When I spend my breaks walking or doing things the movement isn't allowing my vestibular functions to settle. That means I've been getting a lot of extra fatigue and dizziness. So gone are spending the breaks from work on the bike or gardening. And my 10-minute breaks should be sitting still doing nothing – boring and ho hum but oh well. Have you ever tried sitting still and doing nothing for 10 minutes?

One exciting note is that I have another MRI booked this month, I think it's my fourth now. The ABI clinic has requested it as they are looking further into the contusion they found. This one will include the injection of some contrasting dye to highlight the blood vessels in the brain. Never had one of those before so another new experience to chalk up.

The new pills are going ok. Another slight increase in the dosage this week so another week of extreme drowsiness and trippy dreams or nightmares! Plus, I suddenly go out like a light in the evening.

Next month means I will have reached the sick pay limit and need to go onto benefits. Can't believe I've had twenty-eight weeks of sick leave already! I've had to spend the week sorting the doctors and bureaucracy. The Employment and Support Allowance form and online help guides weren't really designed for people struggling with brain injury. In the end I called the helpline, went through it all there and then, so my claim is settled. One task down, next week will mean sorting the tax office.

In the last bit of fun before I sign off, we spent the weekend dog-sitting for our friend's new puppy. Ash was pretty captivated playing with her and snapping loads of photos. It reminded us just how much we love dogs – and how much we hate poo on the floor. So, a fun day, but glad to give her back. She isn't quite three months yet, so swung from a bundle of manic joy to anxiously demanding a lap to curl up in. Bit like me on these pills!

My moods had been changing dramatically for over a year. It wasn't until I started recording the dizziness and fatigue that I realised how closely my emotions tracked them. My mood spiralled down when I became tired, and crashed whenever a dizzy migraine returned. Being able to spot the symptoms helped, as I was able recognise the emotion as a reaction to the dizziness or pain.

Recognising that my dizziness was causing the fear and anxiety was the first step to solving the problem. Being able to take that extra step back helped to show me that the fear wasn't a problem with me, it was a symptom of what I was going through. That little change in perspective meant I could look at my list of tasks without that sense of being overwhelmed or panicking.

Diary entry

FRIDAY: It's odd, these days I feel a little looser, like I'm not trying to force changes and am just letting life flow by. Should that worry me? Am not sure. Surely being relaxed is better. Certainly, I feel better when I feel like I'm not struggling or fighting against something all the time. It's far more relaxing to just let things be. I still fear that I will just coast and let things happen. But that fear is much less now, perhaps because I feel more in control and more appreciative of things when I'm only focussing on a few tasks at a time. It's amazing how much I have done today. Managed to fit in exercise, errands and vocational homework. Yes, I was exhausted by the end of all of that and had a pretty good half hour nap. But I see that as proof that I am getting better. Not long ago I was needing two-hour naps just to get through the day. So, another reminder to slow down, and that I'm getting better. I must work on the pacing part of Fatigue Management. Perspective, Priorities, Planning, Pacing. Sorting out these four things will help me get back on track. Doing what the doctors tell me?! Good heavens, next thing you know I'll be getting better!

The progress was heartening, but I still felt vulnerable out in the world. The busy underground trains and stations were both familiar and frightening territory. My dizziness was fading, but those months of pain had left scars of association. Despite my efforts, I still feared being around crowds and fast-moving vehicles. I treated these fears with the same remedy as dizziness, I practised exposure therapy.

In the early days this meant taking a seat on the bus and watching the world go by. I wasn't moving, I was in crowds but in a safe environment. But still I found a way to worry. *Not the seats at the top of the stairs or near the door, people getting on or off might hit me. If someone sits behind me, I need to move, they might hit me too.* Of course, no one hit me. Over weeks of being ignored by other people who were also just getting through their days, my worries slowly dissipated.

Buses took ages though, just getting to the hospital meant a 90-minute round trip if the appointment was anywhere near rush hour. So, a 10-minute appointment after 20 minutes in the waiting room actually meant I was out and about for two hours. Dealing with all the motion, the busyness and the fears, was exhausting.

But it worked, and after a month I was comfortable with being out. I upped my game and tried taking the tube part of the way. *Bus to the station, tube into the centre, 5-minute walk to the hospital. Then just the reverse on the way back.* If it worked, my round trip could be less than an hour and my fatigue would shrink to match. I was excited and hopeful. *You've planned carefully, you can do this!* The outside world always had a way of intervening though.

Diary entries

FRIDAY: On the way home from my hospital appointment this afternoon, a man smiled at me as we negotiated the crush of a tube elevator. I flashed a small smile back and dismissed the moment. Then I realised he had boarded the same bus and chose to stand opposite my seat. He smiled again. I put my sunglasses on and pretended not to see him mouthing 'I love you'. When I got off at my stop, he was a step behind. He dropped back but followed me round the corner and again into another street. I was freaked by now, but still questioned my judgement. So, I called Ash who agreed it was odd. 'Don't go into our street, go to the church on the other corner. There will be people there.' There were, and the man stopped following me. I walked around the block a few times to be sure.

What the hell is going on? This never happened before, and now two men have threatened me within a few months. Is it that I'm scared and they can see it? The predator sensing the vulnerability of its prey? Damn it! I'm tired and fed up. Fed up with being anxious about my brain. Fed up with not knowing what to do. Fed up with arseholes attacking or stalking me in my own neighbourhood. Fed up with trying to get better and always ending up tired, or emotional or scared – or all three. I've had it! Do I just give up on everything and sink onto the couch in defeat? I know I'd loathe that, well, I'd loathe myself and the feeling that I'd given up. I don't want to stop trying to be normal but sometimes it is just so damned hard.

WEDNESDAY: MRI scan day, it was the one where they inject you with dye. What a horrible feeling the dye gives you. Even through the docs warned me of it I still felt like I'd pee'd my pants. The humiliation and shame of a grown woman feeling that was just awful. Fortunately, the doctors are professional – they must deal with people who feel like that every day. But all the poking with the needle, slapping of veins and the need to hold the wrist in a contorted position to avoid any pain for what seemed like hours. There's a decent bruise forming on the wrist already. I felt really drowsy afterwards so had to cancel another evening with friends. And I'm sad, and Ash has gone out without me. After such a sh*te year I couldn't ask him to stay in with me. Think I'm missing my old social butterfly self. Still I'm getting better. B*llocks to the weight loss, I need comfort food.

Summary of emails with parents

ME: I'm not sleeping well lately. For a change, it is worrying about other people's problems which is keeping me up. I've spent a lot of time this week talking to a friend. She's going through a hard time and I know it is good to be an ear for her to work things through. But worrying about her problems has been keeping me awake and meant today was a write off. This evening, I got a call to say that my friend's worries were over and did I want to join them for a drink. I really did, given how much I'd owned the feelings too, but dealing with them had completely worn me out.

MUM: Did I tell you about the psychiatrist and the pen? The psychiatrist spent most of a session listening while the client lists all their worries over the problems other people were facing. When the list was finally over, the psychiatrist silently held out a pen. Her client looked at it and took it.

'Why did you take that?' The psychiatrist asked.

'I don't know, I don't even want it.'

'If you don't want it then don't take it. It is the same with other people's problems. You don't have to take them on. You can acknowledge the problems and sympathise, but still leave the feelings with them.'

Chapter 10

Vocational rehabilitation
Work, once more, with feeling

June: Fifteen months after the incident

I had lost count of the number of times I'd tried to return to work only to slink away in dejected dizziness. The six months immediately after the incident had been punctuated by fleeting moments of normality, desperate attempts at joining in around the water cooler and, finally, the admission that I needed yet more time. But now, fifteen months after the incident and nearly eight months since my last foray into the office, I had a plan to follow.

Summary of emails with vocational rehabilitation therapist

THERAPIST: How are you getting on with all the things I left you with last week? I know we covered an awful lot in one session. Please find attached a draft letter I have written for your manager. Have a look at the letter and let me know if I have missed anything or made any mistakes. Remember, you are the expert of your condition and job role!

ME: The letter said that the amount of time spent at work will increase in duration every fortnight. But it left the nature of the work duties quite open. I was wondering if those tasks will increase in difficulty every fortnight too or will increase be based on how I cope? Last week I managed to complete an hour of work every day. As you asked, this hour was split into twenty-minute intervals and the tasks were a mix of writing emails and reading documents. Most of it felt ok, but think I will do smaller forays into the inbox as it did bring on the stress symptoms a little. The breaks I had were only five-minute ones so I will make sure I have ten-minute breaks as suggested in your letter. I hope to still fit those in despite the demands of the vestibular physiotherapy exercises.

THERAPIST: Brilliant work on doing an hour a day of computer-based tasks! Ideally, we would want to aim for you to be tolerating at least two hours of computer-based work, with breaks, in a quiet environment before considering a return to the office. For your next appointment, please write out a list of things that trigger your symptoms and what helps to alleviate them. When we meet, we can use that to assess your work duties and create a hierarchy of how stressful you find them. This will help us and your manager to ensure that both your tasks and hours are graded appropriately when you return to the office. And it will help your employer to set up a space for you to work in which might help with the symptoms.

Clinic homework: Vocational rehabilitation

> **Trigger:** Noise, crowds and strobing lights. **Alleviated by:** Removing self from trigger.
> **Trigger:** Interruptions and multiple tasks. **Alleviated by:** A quiet space and time to think something through.

Email to parents

ME: Hope you don't mind that I didn't write last week, but I'm not good when the temperature is over 30 Celsius. The big news is that the vocational rehabilitation clinic have cleared me for a graduated return to work! I will start in a fortnight with two mornings a week in the office. It is exciting and a bit nerve-wracking as I'll still have to fit in all the vestibular exercises and clinic appointments. But I have to try again sometime.

The vocational rehabilitation therapist gave me some interesting homework this week. She said that my colleagues are likely to ask about my absence and recovery. So, alongside the usual 'work strengthening sessions', she asked me to prepare responses for the obvious questions. She wants me to think about how much or how little I want to tell them. The rehabilitation team noted that I don't have to tell them anything at all; it is my business, not theirs. But it is only natural that some people will be curious or concerned. She said that it would help to prepare so I don't feel put on the spot or say any more than I'm comfortable with. I'm really glad she mentioned it, as it simply hadn't occurred to me. I have been through so much, I'm not sure I want to share it all!

The vocational rehabilitation team have written to Alder, my manager, about my return. He is arranging for a small room to be set aside for me to work in. It will double as my work space and, as no-one else is in the room, my quiet space to retreat to. Alder also told me that the HR team are starting a claim with their insurer over my injury. There is scope for the business to receive compensation for the sick leave payments, and for me to return to the salary and benefits I was on before the incident. If that comes through, it would certainly mean the financial worries would be eased.

Speaking of financial worries, my employment sick pay finished last month. At the same time, I applied for government benefits. In typical government fashion, the confirmation came through on the day I had to call them with my clearance for a graduated return. Apparently, I'll get my first and last benefit payment next week as I go back to work the week after. Six weeks to start paying you but less than a week to cancel. Meanwhile, Ash was job hunting after the shambles of the previous employer. There is a process to go through to claim for his back pay but I've no doubt it will be made as torturous as possible. Thank heavens he has landed a new job; I don't know how we'd have coped otherwise.

Diary entry

MONDAY: A busy day and tonight's headache tells me that I've pushed through & over done it. Fitting in three hour-long sessions of the vestibular physiotherapy exercises was exhausting enough, but the vocational rehabilitation homework has been bumped up to six sessions in advance of the return to work next week. Nine hours of therapy, it's longer than a day in the office! In amongst all that was a GP appointment as I needed to sort the return to work and the sick notes with her. We also discussed the trippy pills. I'm aware that the pills could really become a crutch, but need to get to a point where I can do a full day without them. GP agreed but pointed out that this is a question for when I'm back at work, am social again and can manage a full week of both. It is nice to realise that future is achievable. I'm no longer asking those questions: 'will I be like this forever?' or 'what if I'm not able to do the things I want?' I must hold onto this feeling of 'I'll get there, take it easy and don't beat yourself up' on those days when it all just feels a hopeless struggle. There is always hope.

July: Sixteen months after the incident

First day back at work on graduated return

The receptionist was new. I hadn't anticipated that. All my planning: the testing of the commute, making lists of what to say and do, ironing my best shirt twice; none of it had prepared me for a new face guarding the front desk. I hesitated by the door but he had seen me and opened with a professional 'Good morning.'

'Umm, hi.' *Who are you?*

'Can I help you?'

'Umm, Alder. I'm here to…' *To pick up the pieces of my career.*

'Alder Blackman? Do you have an appointment?'

'Sort of, yes.' *I work here. Only I don't. Only I do.*

'Please sign in and I'll call him now.'

I gave in and signed the visitor's book. *I guess that's what I am now.* I'd started work in the building ten years earlier, but all these months away made me a stranger. *I've been so wrapped up in my own life, of course everyone else has moved on too.*

And so it proved. Alder had cleared his morning to escort me round the building. As he introduced new colleagues and familiar faces, I felt even more like an interloper. Everyone had changed. It wasn't just the new employees, change was everywhere. There were promotions, absences, different haircuts, diets of varying success, new babies and deeper wrinkles. It was sobering and surreal.

And I wasn't the only one who felt awkward. Some people hugged, others hung back. We were all trying to work out where I fitted in now. Questions hung in the air, unspoken behind what was said:

'You look great!' *Why don't you look different?*

'It's good to have to back.' *Where have you been?*

One colleague just asked 'What the hell happened?' Thanks to the list in my pocket, that was the easiest to deal with.

'It took a year but I finally got into the neurological clinics – about five of them now. They found a bruise or something in my brain and are all busy working out what happened and what I can do now.'

'God! You must have had a hell of a year.'

'Yeah, it's been… Well, it's been sh*t.'

That was about as open as I felt I could be about what had happened in the last year. But at the same time that was ok. I was back but still recovering so it wasn't a case of 'all sorted, back to normal.'

There were other clues which made it clear to my colleagues that I wasn't magically fixed. My previous role as team manager was being temporarily filled by a colleague who would stay in place for now. Team manager was a demanding full-time role, one that simply wasn't possible when working only two mornings a week. Instead, I had a floating brief where I picked up projects for the department. I was working on my own in a separate room, not returning to a desk in the open plan office.

I was only in the office for two hours, but it was exhausting! I made it home for a late lunch and a nap. That evening I managed to do my vestibular physiotherapy exercises before collapsing into bed for a sixteen-hour sleep. I wasn't back to normal but I'd made it back to the office!

Diary entry

FRIDAY: I've noted before that the need to catch up on a few days' worth of diary entries is a sure sign that I am struggling. Yesterday started with a phone call to the parents as they have been emailing a lot and are worried about my return to work. It was good to talk to them but I needed a nap when we were finished. It couldn't be a long one though as I needed to be in the office that afternoon. It was the second office visit on the graduated return. I saw a few more people and finally sorted everything in the separate room allocated to me. Most of my two hours were spent throwing out papers and files which had seemed important all those months ago. The team had swept everything from my desk into a set of drawers and kept it in the corner, like a wee shrine. It was touching, though meant I also needed to throw out boxes of expired cereal and biscuits. Fortunately, I hadn't left any fruit there. The plan is to do another two mornings next week and increase to three mornings for a fortnight. Then I'll be back at the vocational rehabilitation clinic in early August for new instructions. I'm trying not to get caught up in it all, I already feel the tug of the pace in an office. It would be easy and dangerous to get swept up and crash again. I'm lucky that the project I'm working on is self-contained. But next week there is a meeting taking up all of one morning and a need to sort HR out so I suspect there won't be any work done until the third week. But it is great to be back, really pleasing to feel up for it again. Ash has noticed that I've been a bit more tired but said he is proud of me for getting through the last year and getting back to work. Really nice to hear. Joy is in the simple things.

Summary of emails with employer HR team

HR: I checked with the insurance company this morning and they are awaiting a report directly from your GP. Please ask your GP to arrange this as soon as possible. If you have any medical evidence such as occupational health reports and letters, can you please let me have them. Hope things are improving.

ME: Please find copies of my two latest sick notes, one of which has the planned graduated return to work. The insurance forms you need me to fill in have arrived this week. I'm awaiting another GP appointment so I can confirm release of my medical records. I'll update you as soon as that happens.

Email to self

ME: Double check that all working, holiday and time in lieu days are correctly recorded. Then send the records to HR along with the eight attached sick notes.

While I was only in the office two hours a week, I'd spend hours arranging reports with my GP and releasing medical records to the insurance company. There were pages and pages of forms and I even arranged for diary entries to be released too. Anything I could add to the evidence for loss of earnings for both myself and the company was included.

August: Seventeen months after the incident

Diary entry

THURSDAY: Have to catch up on diary entries so been struggling again. I'm now in the office on Mondays, Wednesdays and Fridays. I'm supposed to only work half a day but leaving the office on time after four hours is impossible. There are always last-minute emails or people stopping me on the stairway with 'just one more thing'. Of course, I'd never remember it so have to go back up to the room and write it down before trying to leave again. Bussing to and from the office is better for the vestibular system and means I avoid the crush and noise of the trains. But a round trip takes three hours. So, four hours in the office actually means seven hours of being out in the world. The vestibular physiotherapy exercises take up another two hours each day and I still have several hospital appointments every week. I try to schedule appointments on days when I'm not in the office so I can rest a bit more.

But even those days are being filled with claim forms. The employment insurance claim is not going smoothly and trying to juggle that between the government demands for an explanation of my short benefit window is really sapping my energy. Sadly, the benefits office don't provide a reason code for: 'I only got one week of payments because you took so damned long to process the form!' Fitting everything in is not easy and it is always the rest breaks that suffer or get missed. Last night I only just managed it all but it was a late night so was a little abrupt with Ash. I do hate doing that, focusing on and having time for everything but the most important person. Will have to change that and work on getting the balance right. Because I am a bit out of whack at the moment. And today was the result. Fourteen hours of sleep interrupted by horrid trippy dreams. They gave way to a dizzy day but I managed to drag myself into hospital for the vocational rehabilitation appointment.

Clinic notes: Vocational rehabilitation

The patient's graduated return has increased to working half a day, three days a week. She reports that she is struggling to stick to timers and to stop working once the set hours are over. She is currently using annual leave to cover days when break-through symptoms mean she is not able to work. These break-through symptoms are likely caused by the patient trying to push through her fatigue rather than taking cognitive breaks. The patient seems to be having trouble with the pacing aspect of Fatigue Management. Priorities are set and a structure is planned. However, the patient does not pace herself to match.

She was reminded to take a 10-minute break every 45 minutes and to ensure that the breaks do not involve moving, reading, talking or 'switching screens'. The patient was reassured that doing a meditation lesson or listening to music, without lyrics, was a suitable cognitive break. During the appointment, we assisted the patient with setting out her graduated work hours for September. She was instructed to construct a new Fatigue Management Planner to match and encouraged to use her timers. She was reminded that, while she might not feel the need for a cognitive break, she will still need one.

Diary entries

WEDNESDAY: I realised this morning that I forgot to take the trippy pill last night as I was out at tai chi. Missing one therapy because I'm busy with another! So had the pill this morning and asked to work from home as negotiating city streets on those pills isn't safe. Managed an hour of work before the pill knocked me out and it was back to bed again. I was able to work in the afternoon but have needed longer breaks than usual. Been a bit delicate all day with dizzy spells from the reading.

FRIDAY: A long day and feeling wiped out. Been trying to keep myself up in the evenings in hope of a getting better sleep with less dizziness. The lack of sleep last night meant I was up early, so just went into the office before everyone else. Felt quite poorly all day so definitely still struggling. I sat in a meeting for ages rather than leaving when my silent alarm went. I'm sure they would understand but it is hard not to feel rude when walking out. I just kept going so I got quite dizzy and unwell and ended up stumbling out anyway. By then I was too unwell to notice any stares. Bonus?!

SATURDAY: Another morning, another difficult night of not sleeping. Then I discovered at breakfast that I had missed another anti-dizzy pill. Really annoying as I was hoping to get to Laurel's party. But between the soporific effect of taking the pill, the dizziness of not having taken it last night and a massive headache, I couldn't get to Laurel's place. Another friend let down. Another weekend written off. My work hours increase next week, I hope I can do this!

September: Eighteen months after the incident

Tweet

Chuffed! Just completed my first full day of work in 18 months. Slowly but surely getting back things!

Diary entry

WEDNESDAY: A very long day and quite a difficult one in the office. I'm so tired that it was a struggle to keep moving, to keep putting one foot in front of the other. I'm having those odd intrusive dreams again, the kind where you wake drenched with sweat and a sense of menace but no idea why. I had been warned about those with the pills and thought

I was through them but no luck. They really are horrid, it is like my imagination has just run away and I can't stop it. Dreamt that I was on a caravan holiday with the brother. We were trapped inside by torrential rain and he was hungover & grumpy. In all, it was a bit of a relief when the dream changed into a zombie invasion. Still vivid and disturbing though and I woke up full of dread quite a few times. Wonder if that is another migraine sign? Either way, my head was groggy so had a slower start to the morning than planned. I managed the vestibular exercises before realising I was late for work. Rushed off to the bus and tried to let the dizziness fade. Of course, it didn't work and I was still dizzy when I made it to the office, only an hour late. Tried to make progress on one of my projects but was interrupted by a colleague. They were letting off steam over one of the latest problems. It was a bit of a shock to the daily structure and the dizziness and headache took a turn for the worse due to the stress. An extra-long break helped me to realise that I can't actually help the team. There is nothing I could do, even if I was well enough. The pause for thinking time helped me to accept that it is a mess I can't clean up. The headache and dizziness were better after that, but still hung around meaning I was a little out of it for the rest of the day. Am aware my limited ability to multi task at the moment might be mistaken for grumpiness. But I'm doing my best!

Email to Alder

ME: We spoke yesterday about the fact that the last week or two have been quite a struggle for me. The vocational rehabilitation team advised that I work just the three days again this week before adding the extra half day. Hopefully this consolidation will help, and I will ask if there is anything else I can do about the dizziness & fatigue when I see the vestibular physiotherapy team next week.

Email to parents

ME: My graduated return to work has had a few setbacks. Basically, I've been running round like an excited puppy just let off the leash as I've been away from the office for 18 months. Today was another vestibular physiotherapy appointment and the docs have reined me in again. One way of doing that was to set even harder exercises to retrain my balance system. They keep reminding me that the only way to fix dizziness is to do things that make you dizzy on purpose so you gain more resistance to it. Not much fun I assure you.

I didn't like having to tell the manager and my team that I needed to slow down again. But they have been brilliant and said 'don't care how long it takes, just want to get you back to full speed eventually'. Alder said he didn't mind if I tell him after the fact when I take holidays so long as I don't put anyone else out over meetings etc. I'm working from home tomorrow, which removes the dizziness and fatigue from the travel – a huge relief! When I next see the vocational rehabilitation team, I'll ask about extending my graduated return timetable. Fortunately, I also see the dizzy docs again so will look at increasing the dosage of the trippy pills.

Some slow days booked in to the Fatigue Management Planner now and everything seems a bit calmer. Last week, my friend said that I'm already much more 'fluid' in conversation than when he saw me three months ago. It is such a relief to know there is always progress even if I don't see it. Suddenly the evening is here and it is time to get ready for another day of work – so pleased to be able to write that!

Chapter 11

Results of the brain scans

A voicemail diagnosis

August: Seventeen months after the incident

In the middle of August, in the middle of a meeting, I missed a phone call from the hospital.

Voice message from the Adult brain injury clinic

> Just to say that your scan from April was discussed in the vascular meeting. It looks like you might have a cavernous haemangioma, and the team agreed they will reconvene once they have the results of your contrasting MRI scan. Here is the number to call, if you have any questions.

If I have any questions? You bet I do! What is a cavernous haemangioma? Which part of the brain is it in? How did it get there? Is it stable? Growing? Shrinking? Did it cause all the problems? Are we doing the right thing to fix it? Will I need surgery? Will this happen again…?

So many questions and a new flood of anxiety because of a 30-second voice message. I returned the call within an hour and reached a receptionist. Most of the team were now on holiday, and the rest weren't available. My number was taken, and I was promised a call back. She assured me there was also a letter in the post which would answer my questions.

Another frantic call to my dad. As a retired GP, he was able to provide a few answers: 'A cavernous haemangioma is a small tangle of weakened blood vessels in the brain. It's just the kind of thing that would bleed after a blow to the head. Or it might have been caused by the injury. Let's hope they call back with more information.'

I tried to control my fears and impatience. More waiting for phone calls. More waiting for a wary postman. More waiting for answers. The promised call and letter never arrived. I did, however, find answers in a letter from another clinic which turned up six weeks later.

September: Eighteen months after the incident

Clinic letter: Neuro-otology/dizzy docs

The patient reports that, since starting the amitriptyline for migraine prophylaxis, her vertigo symptoms have almost stopped. She is on a very low dose and still has some breakthrough symptoms with associated headaches. Exacerbating factors include increased strain from a graded return to work, and attempting to perform some of her vestibular physiotherapy exercises. With regards to the latter, she has found these useful overall but difficult to complete. We recommend that she increases the dose of amitriptyline, as the usual maintenance dose is double her current dosage.

Damn it! I don't want to increase the dosage, that means more of these horrid trippy dreams. But priority one is getting better and doing what the docs say... fine. I'll increase the dose tonight. The rest of this letter had better have some good news.

MRI of the patient's IAM's and brain has been reported as showing normal anatomy of the inner ear structures, though an area of increased signal heterogeneity is noted in the medial aspect of the posterior left cerebellar hemisphere. This was felt to be compatible with either an area of previous haemorrhage or cavernous haemangioma, though further investigation with CT angiogram showed no signs to suggest an underlying vascular anomaly.

What the hell does that mean? Dr Google to the rescue:

IAM is the internal auditory meatus, also known as the meatus acusticus internus, internal acoustic meatus, internal auditory canal, or internal acoustic canal. It is a canal within the petrous part of the temporal bone of the skull between the posterior cranial fossa and the inner ear.

Yeah, that was no help. Time to call dad again.

'After your first scan went missing, they took a second scan which looked into your ear canals and head. That scan showed there were no broken bones but it did find something in the lower left back of your brain. The third scan with the dye to narrowed it down for them. It looks like a bleed caused by the head injury.'

So, eighteen months and three scans later, we finally had proof of a brain bleed. It was a huge relief. At last there was physical evidence of what I had suffered all this time. But I was also frustrated that the diagnosis had taken so long. *Has more damage been done in that time?*

It was a fruitless question as, ultimately, there was no way to tell. That didn't stop me from worrying. But now we had a diagnosis. Solid proof of what had happened in my brain.

Diary entry

SUNDAY: It has been a difficult weekend, I think because I have been putting too much pressure on myself to 'be normal'. Yesterday I woke with a dizzy feeling but forced myself up and off to watch River FC's game. I didn't enjoy that much as had a cracking headache and left early. Another reminder that I can't just force my way through cognitive fatigue. Came home to discover that my tree has gone! The neighbours have cut down the tree which has been my companion through all those long hours in bed. The view leaves me desolate now, there was a lot of emotion invested in that bark. I have spent so many hours alone just looking at the tree that I felt like we were teammates, working together on getting better. Looking out the window at the forlorn stump seems like a horrible metaphor.

Summary of email from Citizens Advice

ME: Further to our telephone conversation, your case will be heard in the Magistrates Court. Please find attached a map of the building for your information.

Diary entry

TUESDAY, THE DAY BEFORE COURT APPEARANCE: A pounding headache last night but I did manage to get to sleep eventually. After waking countless times in the night, I have felt tired and 'on edge' all day. Not helped by the approaching court appearance. Today I watched the video of the assault again so it wouldn't be a shock in court. It didn't leave me feeling as bad as I'd feared but it has meant for a stressed afternoon. Will be glad when tomorrow is over.

My day in court began early. Fear of what lay ahead kept me awake and I watched a hot late-summer dawn build through a crack in the curtain. My brother collected me and we arrived at the courthouse slightly early. We'd had plenty of experience of various hospitals and clinics but very few encounters with the law. A Victim Support officer met us and took us to a small waiting room. Even before nine am it was already stuffy, the smell of stale sweat clung to the worn carpet.

'We'll call you when they are ready for you.'

'Do you know when that might be?'

'The police officer will speak first, and then you'll be called in. Probably a 30-minute wait.'

After she left, I settled onto a thinly padded chair while my brother tried to open a window. Time ticked away loudly as we took turns to shuttle back and forth to the door, checking we hadn't been forgotten about. Thirty minutes' wait turned into an hour so we asked the liaison about the delay.

'We're still waiting for the accused to turn up.'

'I thought he was back in prison for parole violations.'

The liaison looked puzzled and glanced at her notes. 'Umm.'

'Wait, has he been out?' My brother sounded alarmed, then I realised I was too. The man who attacked me could have been following us this very morning. *Does he know where I live?*

'I can't discuss that. His lawyer is here, so it shouldn't be too much longer.'

That was hardly reassuring. 'He's kept everyone waiting, will this count against him in court?'

'I can't discuss that. It shouldn't be long now.'

The clock ticked away another 30 minutes while we waited uneasily on the thin chairs. The liaison popped her head into the room.

'Just to let you know the case is still pending.'

'Has he turned up yet?'

'Just help yourself to more tea.'

I called Alder: 'It doesn't look like I'll make that meeting this afternoon.'

'Take the day off.'

More annual leave used up in anonymous waiting rooms. Eventually we got word.

'The case has started.'

'He's turned up then?'

At her nod my brother asked 'Will the magistrates take into account that he was over two hours late?'

The liaison spoke to me instead. 'The officer is presenting his case now. You'll be called in after that.'

'Can I stay with my sister?'

She couldn't ignore that. 'You can go in with her, but she will be in the witness box. You can sit in the gallery.' The liaison turned back to me. 'We suggest that the victim leaves after giving testimony.' *Victim, that's what she sees in me.*

Whoever thought up the layout of a court room didn't think of it from a witness's point of view. My brother was consigned to a bench at the back of the room, the only supportive face sent to the far periphery of my view. The three magistrates were also distant, seated behind a large desk which loomed over the right-hand side of the witness box.

Straight ahead, impossible to avoid and watching my every move, was the man who had attacked me. I had last seen him cursing and spitting in rage as I swallowed my own blood. He was now freshly washed and tidily dressed. *Hair still wet from a shower; he hasn't been waiting in a hot room for hours.*

Only his lawyer and a small wooden railing stood between us. Of course, he wouldn't try anything in a courtroom, but it is one thing to know that, and quite another to feel safe while being displayed on a raised platform. He didn't speak, but watched closely while I described what had happened. I was desperate not to appear intimidated, grinding my feet into the floor so I couldn't flee. I silently repeated the Victim Support officer's advice: 'Keep looking at the magistrates, tell your story to them' *And ignore the cold creeping up your spine. Just keep standing, just keep talking.* I finished by recounting the walk home and calling the police. His lawyer rose. *Why does he get a lawyer? Wait, should I have a lawyer? I'm doing this all wrong!*

'Why did you throw a spoon at my client?'

'I didn't throw it. He dropped it out of the car and I dropped it back in.'

'How do you "drop" an item into a car? You must have thrown it at him.'

'I'm taller than the car window. I held out my hand and dropped it.'

'When you threw it, it hit him on the head and angered him.'

'I didn't throw it, I dropped it.'

'How does that work?'

'Gravity.'

Out of the corner of my eye I could see my brother shift in the gallery. He was right, I was scared and vulnerable which made me facetious. I was also tired, I'd slept poorly, full of fear about this very moment. Then we'd waited for hours in a hot room while the man who attacked me had slept in and now hid behind his lawyer.

'My client admits to being angry, but all the alleged injuries were in self-defence.'

'Are you serious? Look at him! He is bigger and taller than me.'

'He felt attacked when you threw things at him.'

'I didn't throw anything, I dropped a plastic spoon in the window and kept walking. He then leapt out the car and followed me down the street shouting and spitting.'

'And once you were both on the street, you confronted him.'

'Someone was following me down the street shouting about punching me. I didn't confront him, but I didn't want to be attacked from behind. So, I turned around.'

'To face him?'

'To face him.'

'And that is when you lashed out at him.'

'No, I never attacked him.'

'How can you be sure?'

'I was carrying two heavy shopping bags. My hands were full. I couldn't have attacked him for the same reason that I couldn't defend myself when he threw his punch.'

'He punched you?'

'Yes, as I just said now, and as I told the police on the day and as I state in the video I took at the time while he was trying to throw off the witnesses and attack me again. He got out of the car. He followed me down the street. He shouted all the abuse. **He punched me**. He was not acting out of 'self-defence' because I did **not** attack him.'

Silence filled the court. My attacker shifted. The lawyer cleared her throat.

'You are on long term sick leave, are you not?'

'I was off work then, with a brain injury, but am now back at work. Or I was hoping to get there this afternoon.'

My brother leaned forward. *Fine, I won't get angsty.*

'And, your, ah… illness, does that affect your movement?'

'It's a brain injury, after a football match. I've been open about that with the police and with my filings to the court. The medical notes show that my movements have been impaired for the year leading up to the attack.'

'And does your condition cause any movements, involuntary perhaps, which might be seen as a threat?'

'I get dizzy from time to time but that just makes me weak and fall down.'

'No lurching or sudden movements?'

'Nothing that might cause someone to believe that a person smaller than them, weighed down with a back pack and heavy shopping bags might be about to attack them, no.'

The lawyer looked at her notes and then up at the magistrates' bench. 'My client admits to being angry. But any injuries this woman sustained were out of self-defence.'

Liar! I shook my head and tried to protest. The magistrate cut me off and asked the lawyer if she had any more questions for me.

'No, thank you.'

The magistrate glanced at me. 'Thank you, you can go now.'

The police officer had watched from the gallery and joined my brother and I outside the court room. 'That was brilliant, well done.'

I was relieved, angry and too exhausted to say anything. My brother stepped in and asked about would happen next.

'We usually recommend that the vic... that you don't stay after giving your testimony. I take it you will leave together?'

'Yes, she needs a sit down and some food.'

'Somewhere neutral, somewhere you don't go often?'

'Yes.'

'Good.' The officer turned back to me. 'I'll call this afternoon and let you know.'

We left the building and walked toward the bus stop. My brother stayed close and was looking behind us often. 'The bus stop is ahead.' I told him. 'But, what are you...?'

'Checking who is here, seeing who is around.'

'What?'

He didn't answer, only flagged down an approaching bus.

'That's not our bus.'

'Yes it is, get on.'

He ushered me into a seat before explaining. 'We, I mean Mum, Dad and I, we've talked about this. This guy has done time for violence before. We don't want him or his mates knowing anything about us.'

'I know that. So?'

'So, I was looking to see who was around and if we are being followed.'

I felt cold, and stupid. *Of course. That's what the officer was getting at too.* I clutched my bag and whispered. 'Were we followed?'

He cast a quick glance at the kid a few rows back. 'He was outside the courtroom.'

'Oh god.'

'It's fine. We never use this bus and it doesn't go anywhere near our flats. We'll get off and have lunch in some brand-new place we'll never go to again and just wait him out.'

It's not paranoia if others feel threatened too.

That's what we were still doing several hours later when the officer called. 'I can't believe I'm saying this, but he got off.'

The busy cafe shimmered slightly, dizziness threatening again. I gripped the phone tighter, pressing it to my ear as if that would help absorb the news. 'He got off?'

The officer didn't hide the frustration in his voice. 'Apparently the magistrates felt that he was honest because he admitted to being angry. They thought that since he was so honest about his feelings then of course he would have admitted to the assault too.'

'But…. the video, it showed him being held away from me, all his shouting, the threats?'

'They found that it showed there was an altercation, not what caused it or who was at fault. The magistrates decided that, because the witnesses weren't in court, they couldn't decide between your word and his.'

The missing witnesses. The men who refused to speak.

'So without them…' My world lurched sideways, dizziness had broken in. My brother gripped my arm, disbelief in his face. 'Hang on! They found my word to be equally believable as that of a man with previous convictions for violence against women and dishonesty offences?'

The officer's sigh was long and spoke volumes. All the things he wasn't allowed to say. My brother had been listening to my side of the conversation and mouthed 'Appeal!'

'Appeal' I blurted. 'Can I appeal? I mean, that's ridiculous!'

'No, only the person charged can appeal the decision. I'm sorry.'

'So, what? That's it then? He gets away with it?'

'You could try a civil suit, but, again without the witnesses…' The officer trailed off. I felt the weight of all his work, of his colleagues' work. The initial response, tracking down a man on the run, building a case, the disappointment at the end.

'So, that really is it then?' The repetition sounded horribly final.

'I'm afraid so.' After a pause he continued. 'Did you go somewhere busy, is your brother with you?'

'Yes, we are in some cafe, not sure where.'

'Good.'

'Yeah.' I took a deep breath, willed a confidence I didn't feel. 'Yeah, I'll never see that man again. But I'm afraid you will.'

A wry chuckle, 'Yeah, well, you aren't wrong.'

I did all I could. Keep telling yourself that.

'Right then, I guess… um…'

'Yeah.'

As we gathered our things, my brother noticed that our tail had left. The only shadow following us home was fatigue.

Summary of email from parents

ME: You've done very well after several traumatic events, but it is all experience. The verdict doesn't make sense as we know all the facts. Frustrating for you and the police. Disgusting that he got off but how likely would it be that he would have been sentenced as he'd spent that time inside anyway? Not your problem any more. If you think you see him again then pop into a shop or cafe to pass the time. Also, if the insurance money comes through then that will help you to pace out the recovery. After a year out you are planning on pushing your hours at work after a few weeks of slow introduction. However, it will be good to ask the vocational rehab team as they are a good brake and third party to consult. You are looking and sounding so much better than a year ago. You must be pleased at how well you are doing and how much you are managing to do every day now. Though it's good to remember to take time out.

Chapter 12

Therapeutic and diagnostic orders

Much therapy, very wow

October: Nineteen months after the incident

Vestibular physiotherapy exercises

> **Exercise six – Balance:** Static standing: Stand on one leg for 30 seconds. Be sure to practice on either leg. You are now on the hardest level so stand on a cushion with eyes closed and turn head from side to side.

The alarm went off at 12noon: time for second daily set of vestibular physiotherapy exercises. *Already?* It felt like I'd only just recovered from the dizziness brought on by the first set. This morning I had woken slowly with a headache. Despite the groggy feeling I'd managed to do the exercises and endure the accompanying half hour of dizziness before I was well enough for breakfast. But that was a few hours ago and it was time to get dizzy again. If I left it any later, I wouldn't manage lunch until late and then the third set would be late and then dinner…

Ugh, fine. I dragged myself up and reluctantly began to move. The first five exercises went ok, despite the therapist having ramped the difficulty level up to the highest possible. *I hate this.* Only one more exercise to do this round. *Think of the progress you've made!*

Distracted by this thought I lost my rhythm. *Sh*t, I'm falling!* My eyes flew open as the world span under my balancing leg. I tried to grab the table but my flailing hand went wide. *F*ccckkk!* I landed heavily on my knee before instinct kicked in, and I managed to roll through the rest of the landing. Mercifully, my head didn't hit anything. *Thank you, primary school gymnastics!*

The trusty bag of frozen peas was applied to yet another bruise and I sank into a moody afternoon on the sofa. *Damn it, I hate these exercises.* I was heartily sick of vestibular physiotherapy by this point. It wasn't the falling that I hated, this was the first and indeed only time that had happened.

No, the problem was that the exercises brought on the very symptoms I was trying to escape. It felt like I was torturing myself three times a day. A regular schedule of self-inflicted pain. But it was working. I could see the progress. The early exercises had been challenging at first, but now I was doing similar motions daily without triggering any symptoms. The vestibular physiotherapist had been right to increase the difficulty level. But that meant I was back to being tired, sick and dizzy three times a day.

That was bad enough but I also hated the exercises because they set a limit on my other activities. I'd not been to yoga for months because much of my vestibular 'credit' was being spent on these exercises. I'd cut back on so many other things to make time for these exercises that resentment and hatred had set in. I was hoping, really hoping, that when I next saw the vestibular physiotherapist they would declare the treatment complete. *Dangerous thinking, what if I'm told to keep doing them? Then you'll keep doing them because they are working!* I kept on doing the exercises, even after my fall. And I kept on hating them too.

Diary entry

TUESDAY: I realised today that I've had three nights in a row when the trippy pills haven't turned me into a zombie before 9pm. I was in the office yesterday and left with a headache once my hours were done. Despite that, I was surprisingly awake last night. Ash has noticed this trend too so it is definitely an improvement! It didn't last though as I was woozy when the alarm went off this morning. I'd had those horrid dreams again, the ones where you think you are awake but you aren't. This time I woke feeling really thirsty and drowsy so I opened the champagne bottle beside my bed and drank it. Then I woke from that dream and realised that I'd opened the champagne in my sleep and spilt it everywhere. Then I woke up again and realised that of course I don't keep champagne by the bed. Then I actually woke up. It took me a while to work out that I'd had a dream within a dream within a dream within a dream. If that wasn't trippy enough then there were times through-out the day when I'd suddenly think 'wait, am I actually pouring this tea or am I going to wake up in bed in a moment?' I've noticed that these kinds of dreams come when I'm struggling with dizziness and am trying to push through the fatigue. I know the fatigue is worse because of these damned vestibular exercises! But I've boosted them to the highest level I can manage in advance of the appointment so hopefully I'll be able to stop doing them. Time for bed now, woozy again.

Tweet
Hurray, the dizzy exercises have worked! My balance and gaze stabilisation are back within normal ranges! Vestibular physiotherapist says I can stop them and focus on getting life back to normal. And find some fitness :)

November: Twenty months after the incident

Tweet
New research shows that heading a football can result in an impact of 100 gees to the brain! Now you tell me...

Clinic notes: Adult brain injury

Since we last saw the patient, she has commenced a return to work with the support of the vocational rehabilitation team. She is on a graded return and is currently working three days per week. On the advice of the neuro-otology team, her vestibular migraine medication has been increased and will be upped again to the standard base dose. This has significantly helped her headaches and dizziness which have in turn helped with the sleep patterns. The patient has completed a treatment of vestibular physiotherapy exercises and is now working on other forms of balance exercise including cycling and yoga. The patient reports mood and anxiety have improved despite the fact that she is still waiting to be seen by the CBT clinic. The plan from her neurovascular meeting, where her images were previously discussed in view of the suspicions of a bleed, is to carry out a repeat MRI. The patient should see the date for this soon.

Yay, more waiting! In between all the waiting, and the exercises, and the homework and the work, there was a life to rebuild. There had been little time to see anyone but my friends had kept in touch through emails and texts. Finally, towards the end of month, I managed to help at a River FC football training. Hazel, the coach, and Maple were delighted to see me, but there were rules.

'No running! If you need a sit down, just take one. You don't need to explain. You don't have to do anything. But the goalkeeper would really like some coaching time…'

'Yes, I've been promising her that one-on-one session for months. Tonight has been protected in the Fatigue Management Planner for weeks and I've planned out a session for her.'

'Whoop! But no running!'

Hazel had set aside an area at the far end of the training pitch for the goalkeeper and I to train in peace. 'Maple suggested it. She pointed out that we didn't want you to be hit in the head by any stray footballs.'

'It's like you read my mind.'

'The keeper is warming up down there, waiting for you.'

The last time I'd been on a football pitch I was dizzy and terrified. Everything had felt wrong. Since then, I'd had counselling, physiotherapy, advice, a diagnosis and a plan. I'd worked so hard over the last few months and here, on the pitch, I could feel almost normal again. I was elated and it showed.

'Stop running! No running! I'm not explaining to Ash how you hit your head again!'

The keeper and I went through some drills together. I was moving again! Jumping, skipping and, when Hazel wasn't watching, even running a little. I was careful to avoid any possibility of contact so only watched most of the drills. I didn't feel completely fearless, there were still times when the crunch and slap of a hard tackle would make me flinch. I spent a lot of time checking on what the others were doing, making sure I wasn't in any firing lines.

It started raining halfway through training. I took a moment to enjoy the bright scent of wet grass, the salty tang of sweat, laughter in the air, the burn of muscles being used at last. I slowed as the ground became slippery. My movements were checked a little, and not just by the loss of fitness over the last 20 months. But I was there, with my friends again, part of a team. *This is it; this is the reason for all the hard work.*

Maple was also enjoying the camaraderie after her hiatus from the game. We didn't get much of a chance to talk until after the training. As Maple and I walked back to the train station together we caught up on each other's news. Our conversation was interrupted when an ambulance raced past with siren and lights blazing. The flashing blue lanced through the wet night and flickered in a million drops of water. The strobing built until I could see nothing else. I felt myself shut down. There was nothing I could do to stop it. My brain switched off in the middle of a conversation in the middle of a pedestrian crossing.

I could see Maple's face peering into mine, her mouth moving urgently. *She looks worried, wonder what she is saying.* The ambulance had gone, the traffic lights changed. I was still lost. Maple stared down the angry drivers and guided me across the road. Hazel ran back to join us and she and Maple both walked me slowly towards the station as I recovered. It didn't take long to find myself again. But the fact that I could still be that vulnerable in public was terrifying. *What if my friends hadn't been there?*

More fears to try to control but help was on the way. I'd been referred for CBT in March. The adult brain injury clinic had repeatedly said that it would help with my fear and anxiety but the waiting list was proving long. Frankly, there was so much else going on that I'd forgotten about the referral completely. It was a bit of a surprise when I received a call about a cancellation and could I attend clinic the next day?

Tweet

On waiting list ten months and only had given 24hr notice of appt. Work and meetings to rearrange but managed to turn up 30mins early. Fortunately, that gives me time to re-write the Fatigue Management Planner... Again!

Diary entry

TUESDAY: I find myself avoiding the diary and it feels like a chore. But then I'm so tired that I'm seeing everything as a chore at the moment. I realised that I've been clenching my teeth more, damn I hope I don't crack my molars again! This morning started early as I needed to be at hospital by 9am for the initial CBT assessment. Because I was a fill in for a last-minute cancellation my patient file hadn't arrived. This meant that most of the appointment was spent filling in the CBT therapist about the injury and symptoms. The truncated sleep and ever-present fatigue meant that I felt rotten the whole time. I was so tired that I didn't realise how upset I was by events of the past year until the tears began to fall. The therapist was kind, and the appointment ended hopefully – and with yet more homework. On my way out for some breathing space in the park I made way for an elderly couple. Seeing the old man slowly shuffle his way through the hospital foyer really struck me. He could barely move while his wife felt she had to make apologies while asking for a wheelchair. Made me realise I should be counting my lucky stars.

Clinic homework: CBT

CBT is about changing unhelpful habits of thinking. The aim is to help you deal with overwhelming problems in a more positive way by breaking them down into smaller parts. CBT is based on the concept that your thoughts, feelings, physical sensations and actions are interconnected, and that negative thoughts and feelings can trap you in a vicious cycle. We suggest you start by making a thought record the next time you feel overwhelmed. Think about:

1. Triggers: what has happened to make you feel this way?
   Ash is very quiet this evening and seems to be impatient.
2. Negative thoughts: what am I thinking right now?
   He's annoyed with me; I've forgotten something important again.
3. Physical reactions: how am I feeling right now?
   Clenched teeth, anxious, worried, headache, dizzy, scared again.
4. Actions: what can I actually do in this situation?
   Ask him.

It looks so simple when you write it down like that. I couldn't get to that answer by myself. When I did check in, turns out he was brooding on a problem from work. *It has nothing to do with me!* The relief was instant, I stopped worrying, the headache and dizziness and fear all disappeared. *Damn that was easy! I should try it again.*

Email to parents

ME: November is nearly over and I'm only just managing to write, sorry! The last few weeks have been a mix of work and rest. On the recommendation of the neuro-otologists (dizzy docs), I've been upping the trippy pills so am having some very odd dreams again. This is the second attempt at increasing the dose as the first one resulted in odd headaches and fatigue. I had a week of not managing much at all

– more annual leave used up. Tried again and it seems to be going well this time. To celebrate, the vocational rehabilitation team have upped my working hours. Am now trying to do two half and two full days of work a week. At the moment it is going ok, but I've been working from home a lot to avoid the vestibular fatigue of a commute.

CBT is proving interesting but exhausting. I have been doing that through-out November. I've definitely developed habits of unhelpful thoughts and behaviours during this recovery. Lots of energy going into doing their homework and stopping those thoughts at the moment. It's going well but I can't help but think that this would all have been far more helpful if I'd had it closer to the injury on the ninth of March last year.

The docs also want me to keep doing mindfulness and to work on my fitness. So, I managed to get to tai chi for the first time in a while. The teacher pulled me aside to say that the change in me is marked. That I'm much more alert and show more personality than when I started over a year ago. It was really sweet of him to say. He said the change is most marked in the eyes – like I'm awake now. I did enjoy the tai chi but noted that my balance has deteriorated. Time to get the Fatigue Management Planner out again and make sure I fit in time to exercise. Didn't think I'd be doing tai chi, yoga and meditation. Odd the way life turns out sometimes

Diary entry

FRIDAY: I've managed to get to the office for four days in a row for the first time. Granted, two of those days were half days in the office, but I still had to get there! Yesterday was a full day in the office and it really was 'a game of two halves'. The morning was nicely structured with timers to ensure I took breaks. The afternoon meeting was supposed to be half an hour but ended up being nearly two hours. I hadn't set a timer, as thirty minutes is well within my concentration limit. It wasn't until the end that I realised the time that had passed and how ill I felt after missing my hourly breaks. I'd pushed my fatigue again without realising it. Fatigue is falling over everything and numbing me. I'm clumsier too, walking into more things and dropping bits more often. Damn it!

Fatigue is pain
Grinding the gears in the brain
I'm moving in slow-motion
Wading through life

Clinic letter to employer from vocational rehabilitation team

> The patient is currently completing a graded return to work and is grateful for your implementation of this advice as she is very keen to continue her working role. Overall, she has been managing her symptoms of vestibular dysfunction well; however, she reports that she is still suffering from migraines and dizziness. These have recently worsened and exacerbate her other symptoms. The patient is managing this to some extent by taking regular rest breaks at work, however this remains an ongoing issue.
>
> The patient is currently working four days a week, which consists of two full and two half days. She is due to increase her hours on the 30th of November to working four full days per week. Due to the ongoing symptoms it would be beneficial to maintain her current hours until the new year, with a view to returning to full time employment in March 2016.

December: Twenty-one months after the incident

Email to parents

ME: Things are ticking along here. The consolidation of the working hours seems to be helping and I'm a bit more awake again. The vocational rehabilitation team were right to hold back on increasing my hours this month. I'm not as tired as I was a few weeks back so am able to be a bit more social again. Just in time for party season! We had two parties on Saturday. Our friends are heading back down under for good. It was sad and a bit odd to be saying 'right, have a nice rest of your life'. Then it was off to another pub for a birthday party. I was awake and talking to people and feeling very much a part of things rather than just struggling to be there. So that was great, really pleased!

Work is going well at the moment and I'm a lot more relaxed about it now that I've settled into a routine. Something new pops up now and then, as expected when I've been away for this long, but nothing drastic. I did do the classic digging up of a potential massive problem at 4.30 on a Friday. But the beauty of not being in management any more is that is it above my paygrade and I can just email it up a paygrade for others to deal with. I'm still chasing HR for any news on the insurance case though. It's a little frustrating that I seem to be doing all the work on that. Do they not want their pay-out at all? Ah well, can take a horse to water and all that. Despite that frustration, the fact that I'm in a wee office on my own means that my day is much quieter than it used to be. Plus, I'm not dragged into projects or gossip that I don't need to be involved in. As the days turn colder and darker, I'm celebrating having my own heater and window in the office.

At home, the house has been neglected a bit as we both run out of time between work and my hospital appointments and therapies. As we spent more time at home in winter, we got in a cleaning lady to treat ourselves. It means that my plans to work from home today have been disrupted by (in no particular order):

- gas repairmen
- hospital appointments
- a cleaner turning up and bravely going into places trained marines would think twice about
- that awkward guilt caused when someone you don't know is quietly judging you over the state of your kitchen cupboards
- a migraine

Clinic homework: CBT

Incident: on my bike for exercise today and witnessed another cyclist have an altercation. Two pedestrians stepped into the road without looking. Cyclist tried to avoid them but couldn't. No one hurt, but passing cabbie urged the pedestrians to punch cyclist even though it was the pedestrians' fault.

Unhelpful thought: going over and over the incident thinking about the injustice and the threat to me as a fellow cyclist. Actions of cabbie ultimately threatening, wanted to reason with him and defend cyclist.

Balanced thought: I wasn't involved, so a sense of distance helped.

Thinking distortion: personalising, mind reading and jumping to worst-case-scenario.

Lesson: I jump to conclusions when tired, need to pay more attention to my fatigue.

Actions: take more care and time to stop.

Clinic notes: Cognitive Behavioural Therapy

> I have now discharged this lady from CBT. The patient was proactive and has been taught how to monitor and challenge her negative thoughts and to identify thinking errors. I have encouraged her to continue to pace and grade her activities and her return to work. She continues to have goals to work on and is keen to practice and test out behavioural experiments.

Whoop! Another clinic successfully completed! I was getting better at managing my anxiety. It had taken weeks of constant attention to work on the habit. Every now and then I could stop feeding the circle of anxiety that would spiral me down into a depressive mood. That I could now do that was yet more proof of improvement. I was getting better; the treatments were working.

> ### Tweet
> Major milestone in the brain injury recovery today: my first pun in nearly two years.

Email to parents

ME: You can tell things are going well as you get two emails this month! It's already the end of what had been a stupidly warm December in the United Kingdom. We have daffodils out and I spent yesterday watching a football match in a t-shirt! At this time of year, I'm usually head to toe in my various furry garments and in three pairs of leggings. Some very weird weather going on this year and the reports from down under show that it seems to be happening everywhere.

Ash and I are both working up to midday on Christmas Eve, but it is already feeling like the big rush is over. I am still doing two half & two full days of work a week, and it isn't a struggle. The fact that I'm coping with that is fantastic! The calendar has been busy this month but I've managed to get to three Christmas parties too.

I've heard back about my November MRI. Basically, the professors got round a table and discussed me again. They've decided they don't need any more scans for now and I don't need continual monitoring which is great. They'll keep me on their lists for a year and if I get any more symptoms, they'll sort out another scan to check for bleeding. So that is good news! I have a few final appointments in January to wrap up the vestibular physiotherapy and am starting to feel like I'm being allowed out into the world again :-)

Diary entry

NEW YEAR'S EVE 2015: Last day of the year already! And I'm writing this up while also cooking, listening to music and ignoring the noise of the dishwasher. The fact that the brain can do all four things just shows what a long way I've come. Tried to have a nap ahead of the party tonight, but took a while to 'settle'. God, I feel like a toddler sometimes! The fact that I don't just zonk off when I have had the trippy pills is another improvement. Was speaking to the brother on our walk today and we were both saying that we were in good places. Yes, we both have challenges with health and jobs. But we are both in happy frames of mind and not too worried about things. Managing to be in the moment a bit more. It is really nice to be in that mood. Do you have to have had a brain injury or other life changing event to get to that place? Either way, I hope it continues and that we (husband included) can carry that feeling and attitude to the challenges ahead. Time to head to the party – Happy New Year!

2016: Planning

Chapter 13

If it's Tuesday, this must be a migraine

January: Twenty-two months after the incident

Summary of emails with Hazel

HAZEL: I can't do football team training next week. Can you help the team captain if you're about? How's things?

ME: I'll be in & out of hospital with several clinic appointments booked that day so probably won't make training I'm afraid – sorry! Am also starting to do four full days at work which is a bit of a big step but the vocational rehabilitation people say 'if you don't push it you won't improve.'

Diary entry

TUESDAY: The pills are pulling some trippy sh*te and giving me insanely weird nightmares, the 'wake up drenched in sweat & fear' ones again. I wake with vivid after-images, a pounding heart and a feeling of dread. So, I was awake for ages then fell asleep just before the alarm. Busy day in the office and setting the timer for 45 mins on, 15 off seems to be going well. There have been a few times I just carry on as I am right in the middle of something when the timer stops. Home on the train and seem to be getting the knack of public transport again. I'm finding commuting and being out in public a lot easier because I'm not weighed down by fear. I no longer worry about falling or that I might see or hear something that isn't there. Amazing what a difference living with less fear makes. The fear may be rational given the symptoms, but living in it, wallowing in it only held me back. I'm really looking forward to getting on the bike for my commute. All in good time!

Email to parents

ME: The four full days of work went well last week. Though it was damned tiring as I had to fit it in around lots of hospital appointments as my therapies and clinics wrap up. I see the vocational rehabilitation people on Friday and will ask them for a plan to stretch out the return again. Boss doesn't mind how long it takes and I'm in no rush so slower is better. Before Christmas I had a word with the boss about not being in any rush to go back to my old job and things have moved rather quickly since then.

 The current plan is that I'll take back a part time role which I handed off three years ago. The cover brought in will carry on doing my management role, and I'll be back in my old team as an odd bod rather than manager. I'm relatively happy with that. Admit that I'm trying not to see it as a demotion but rather that I get to go back to a more stress-free level of work and stay in the department I like. So that will sort itself out and bed in over the next wee while. There are likely to be retirements in the next few years meaning I should be able to work my way back in to management over two years.

Email to Alder

ME: Good afternoon, I'm afraid my hospital appointment was two hours late this morning but I did manage to edit those documents over the waiting room wi-fi. Ironically, the appointment with the dizzy docs brought on a migraine and I have more hospital appointments tomorrow. Suggest I take holiday today & tomorrow and will be back at work on Monday, hope that is ok? Will get you the forms as soon as possible.

Clinic notes: Neuro-otology/dizzy docs

As you are aware the patient has been affected by migrainous vertigo for which she has been using amitriptyline as prophylaxis. She is now tolerating the standard base dose and this has greatly reduced the number of episodes. However, she is experiencing an increase in side effects due to the increases in dosage. We encourage her to persist at this dose level despite these effects which should stabilise over the next few months. The patient is reporting a struggle to adhere to her Fatigue Management Planner due to the return to work. She needs to persist in her exercises and adhere to her Fatigue Management Planner to help ameliorate the symptoms.

I'm trying so damned hard. Can't you give me a break?

Clinic notes: Vestibular physiotherapy

The patient has attended a course of rehabilitation which focused on maximising her balance, functional gait, gaze stability and visual vertigo symptoms. She is currently working the equivalent of four days a week, is attending tai chi and yoga as well as rebuilding her cycling fitness. The patient has fully achieved all of her rehabilitation goals and is now discharged from our service.

Tweet
Hurray! 22 months after brain injury, my balance & dizziness back to normal so vestibular physiotherapy people are 'releasing me into the wild'. Another clinic down!

February: Twenty-three months after the incident

Tweet
Oh sh*t! I just caught myself shuffling along in my slippers saying 'kids these days'.

The first week of February disappeared in a fog. The entries in my diary are stunted and some were even dated as January. The first month of the year had been so busy that I didn't notice when it ended. The days had flown by in a whirl of hospital appointments, exercise and therapy regimes and the effort of adding an extra day of work every week. I had also taken the advice of the dizzy docs to try new things and picked up the cello for the first time since the incident. I was pushing through the cognitive fatigue again. Sometimes the best thing I could do for my recovery was nothing, but it was so hard to remember.

The graduated return had me working four full days a week. It was exhausting, even though I worked one of those days from home to avoid the commute. I'd also spent a lot of work and personal time on the employment insurance case again. The HR team had asked me to chase it on their behalf. I was learning that people assume I can do more tasks despite working fewer hours. However, I did it, the prospect of a financial settlement to assist my recovery, and my employer's adaptation to it, kept me going. I was adept at leaving messages with receptionists now but my numerous emails and phone calls were again met with unfulfilled promises of a call back.

Given all that, it shouldn't have come as a surprise that a week disappeared, consumed by fog. It was a minor fog though compared to the early days when entire seasons passed by in a grey dash of pain. *I am improving, it is tangible now. I can feel it in the strength of my muscles, the coordination that happens without needing to concentrate and the hours I can spend in meetings without the dizzy lightheaded confusion descending once more.*

The graduated return plan stipulated an increase to 4.5 work days in the middle of February. I wasn't sure if that was a logical step to keep pushing the return or if it was (excuse the pun) a headlong rush into another collapse. Ultimately, I could only try it and see.

Tweet

Two years on from the brain injury and completed my first cycle commute. Yeah baby!

It might sound like a small thing, but the return to a cycle commute helped my recovery in many different ways. I needed to keep exercising my body and vestibular system to avoid dizziness. Commuting by bicycle meant I could fit exercise into my day far more easily. It also meant I no longer bookended my working day by spending hours on destabilising buses or trains. It took a while to build up my cycling stamina again, but being able to spend a commute treating my dizziness rather than triggering it was a boost to my state of mind.

Email to Hazel

ME: I was sad not to watch the game yesterday, but things aren't going so well. The vocational rehabilitation clinic wanted to me to increase my hours by another half day this month and I did. But I'm not sure it has worked as, oh man the fatigue! I'm so bloody tired all the time. Only been up 90 minutes this morning and already need another nap. I'll persist for one more week of working 4.5 days and if I don't feel any better, I'm dropping my hours back. That would mean dropping the vocational rehabilitation team's plan to get me back to full time hours by Easter' goal but hey, this whole recovery has been a game of moving goalposts anyway.

March: Two years after the incident

Diary entries

WEDNESDAY 9TH OF MARCH: Writing that in the diary has given me the third moment today when I've remembered the two-year anniversary of the incident. Oddly, think I remembered it more yesterday. It has been a full-on day, but also my life is getting back together so it doesn't feel like a horrible milestone this year. After I caught up with the parents I headed to work on the bus. Am glad I didn't ride as I left the morning meeting exhausted and woozy. Think I may have said something odd in there, certainly one of the managers looked at me as if I had. It must be clear that I'm struggling. Thankful that Alder readily agreed to reduce the hours. When I'd recovered a little, I finally spoke to the employer's insurance chap. He's had the case for nearly a year but can only advise that we continue to wait. Ugh. Still I'm happy to have been well enough to spend this anniversary working. It is nice to feel that the hard work of the last two years is paying dividends. Yay!

TUESDAY: Woke up to the alarm this morning and had a very thick head. Perhaps I did too much in the office yesterday? Anyway, decided that meant I should probably stay in bed to so I did. Realised I was averse to the bright light so recorded it as another migraine and went back to bed.

TUESDAY: Another Tuesday which didn't go according to plan. I was up and ready to go to the office – except that I felt awful. So, wrote work off for the day, apologised to folk via the work email and moved my days off around to cover it.

TUESDAY: Knew that something was up when I woke after a series of very trippy dreams. And of course, it's a Tuesday again. Given the way I was feeling I sat on the sofa to give myself a rest before getting on the bike, only to wake up over three hours later. So, it was back to bed. Another day written off, another migraine entered into the tracker.

April: Two years and one month after the incident

I knew the place. We'd had drinks there for Perry years before the incident. He'd had a terrible birthday of long work meetings but it was brightened by a cold beer and the woman in red heels at the bar. *Good memory!* I was pleased with being able to recall that, but still lingered across the road. *There is nothing to be nervous about. You've been invited.*

The invitation had arrived out of the blue. The captain of City United would love to see me at her birthday party. I'd managed to fit in half an hour at her birthday two years ago, immediately after the incident. But it was a quick drink in a quiet bar and I didn't remember much about it. *Your fingers gripping the bar, dizziness confusing the barman who mistook it for drunkenness at three in the afternoon.*

Last year, my Fatigue Management Planner was full of clinic appointments, exercises and homework. *Did I even get an invite?* It didn't matter. Here I was, here she was. She had been the only one from City United who had kept in touch for a few months after the incident. *I owe her.* But the others, I'd cried for hours over them. They will be here too. *You owe them nothing.*

I'd made room in the planner for an hour at the party. It wasn't much, but things had been a struggle lately. It was all I felt I could manage. *Say hullo, show your face, a lime and soda and then home again.* It was early but the room was already crowded. I found the captain at the bar.

'You came, great to see you.'

'It's great to see you too. Thank you for the invite. Happy Birthday.'

'How are you?'

'Well…'

A tug on her arm interrupted. 'There's the birthday girl!'

She was wrapped up in a bear hug as half a dozen newcomers drew her slowly away. I ordered my lime and soda and looked around for a friendly face.

'Hullo again.'

'Oh. Hi.' *Who is this guy?*

'It's great to see you again. How are you doing?'

'Umm.' *Just admit it, you have a good excuse for not remembering names.* 'Sorry, I'm having trouble recalling your name. It isn't personal it's just…' *Deep breath, you have this explanation sorted.*

'Is it still your injury?'

'What the…?'

'I'm the captain's friend, Lyndon. We met at this birthday party two years ago, when you had just been hit on the head.'

'I… Wait, you remember that?'

'You were having balance problems and needed to leave but couldn't remember the way. I walked you to the train station then went back to the pub.'

Our feet walking in step, my apologies, his concern. 'I'm sorry, I do remember a little now. Thank you.'

'Weird, we were all worried. I remember it so well.'

'I promise you, it is nothing personal. The whole of 2014 is a vague dream to me.'

'Jesus! Is that why we've not seen you for ages.'

'Yes, lots of neurological clinics, scans, pills, therapies. This is the first time out with everyone again. The doc's have released me into the wild.' It was a weak joke, but he chuckled all the same.

'Your teammates will be happy to see you again.'

'I wouldn't bet on it.' *Damn, I still speak without thinking. Look you've confused him.* Lyndon had been kind to me and deserved an explanation. 'I'm sorry, that sounded bitter. But, well, the rest of the team stopped speaking to me after the injury.'

Lyndon shifted. 'Oh, well. I'm sure they didn't mean to lose touch. It's just life, you know.'

They had plenty of chances. Don't say that. Just admit you must be wrong. 'Of course.'

'I'm sure it's nothing personal. They'll be thrilled to see you again.'

'Of course.' The hollow tone betrayed my true opinion. We watched our respective feet during an awkward pause. A shadow fell over them and I looked up into a face that had been familiar once. 'Cherry?'

I'd known Cherry for years, her name came back to me easily. I'd called it out so many times on the football pitch, in bars and pubs and parties like this one. She stared at me but didn't respond. *Make an effort. Lyndon might be right.* 'Cherry, nice to see you. It's been a while. How are you?'

Cherry's silence felt hard, *the stone in the middle.* Her eyes looked into mine for an age, then she turned to Lyndon. 'Excuse me.'

Confused, Lyndon and I moved back a little. Cherry dragged out a high bar stool then looked at me again. With a sniff, she spun around and sat down. We were cut off from the group, our only view was the back of her head. Cherry hadn't been in contact for over two years but she had managed to acknowledge, deride, dismiss and alienate me within a minute. It was a masterpiece. As was Lyndon's face when he finally breathed. 'Oh. My. God.'

'Well, that felt…brutal.' *This is what happens when you hope.*

'I've never seen anything like that.'

'It might be best if I leave.'

'No, you could…' Lyndon trailed off.

I didn't know what to do either. But I knew what I didn't want to do. *You owe her.* 'Yeah. I'll call it a night. Don't want to, y'know, ruin her birthday.'

The captain was in a middle of a large group. I was wary of causing another scene so slunk out, humiliated. Over the next week, shame turned to anger and stirred up feelings around the behaviour of my old City United teammates which I'd thought I'd dealt with. I spent a stupid amount of time having internal arguments with them again. Fantasy conversations where I'd force people to see how much they hurt me and to inflict guilt in return. It interfered with my recovery for days. Seems I hadn't let go of the hurt and wanted them to see it, to justify the pain they have caused.

But I just had to deal with it. It was clear there was no route open to give me satisfaction or undo the emotions even if everything goes as I desire. What could they say or do to make me happy? A cheap 'sorry'? It wouldn't go back to post-match guffaws in the pub. Those days are just memories now, but memories I'd like to keep unspoilt. To do that, I'll have to let go. Stop trying to control them in a fantasy world. They have moved on, but so have I. *Remember that! I have fought for these last months. I am me again. A new me that they don't know and I have no obligations to them.*

Clinic notes: Vocational rehabilitation

Our intervention has focused on helping the patient to return to work by liaising with her employer and following a graded return to work plan which looked at reduced duties as well as hours. Throughout the course of her graded return to work her job role has changed which means she is no longer a manager and no longer responsible for supervising people. She notes that she is happy with this decision and finds this less stressful. The patient is now managing four days' work a week. She recently tried to increase this by another half day but found that it brought on her symptoms. The patient reports that she still experiences migraines and dizziness, which the amitriptyline pills will assist her with. We are pleased to discharge her from the vocational rehabilitation service.

Tweet
Whoop! Three brain injury clinics down, two to go.

Diary entries: Hazel's wedding

SATURDAY: I was exhausted so took Friday off work to be sure I was fit for the big day. But as soon as I woke up, I knew that I wouldn't make Hazel's wedding. That was upsetting and the frustration and sadness coloured the whole day. I've had a few grumps and a lot of down moments about how I'm progressing. Am questioning if I'm capable of charting my graduated return to work now that I've been discharged from vocational rehabilitation. All in all, a write-off of a weekend which I'd really been looking forward to. Not sure about work on Monday – we'll see.

MONDAY: Nope, getting to the office was not an option today. I managed to get some food this morning and went off to doze in the sun. Surfaced again about noon so had lunch and went for a walk as the brother suggested. That did help, first time I was actually outside since Thursday. Felt well enough to do half a day of work from home, so if I can do the same on my day off this week that will keep me up with the schedule. Took it easy and certainly felt a bit woozy at points but I got a decent bit done. Pleased not to have to use up more annual leave on a migraine.

Tweet

Migraines wrote off last week but I was back into the office and managed a cycle commute each day. So, have ridden 55km! It is the most I've done since the injury over two years ago. Feeling awesome & exhausted...

May: Two years and two months after the incident

Diary entries

SUNDAY: I was determined to make Maple's baby shower this afternoon. It was a loud environment with new people, names to remember, conversations to listen over and I even managed to crack jokes! Really pleased and feeling happy & normal again.

MONDAY: In bed last night the world was spinning for the first time in a while and I had strange, anxious dreams again. So, it wasn't too much of a surprise to find I was still woozy on waking. Another migraine so more apologies to work and took today & tomorrow off. Damn it! I was only out for five hours yesterday but will need two days of annual leave to recover.

Summary of emails with Hazel

ME: Sorry, I won't make training this week.

HAZEL: Ah mate, I'm sorry. Migraines? You managed any work at all? Hope the bank holiday is good to you, see you soon, I hope.

ME: Yeah, had a few migraines in a row. Which means it is probably the same one and I'm not getting rid of it. Used up a fair bit of annual leave on them so hoping for a good weekend.

Diary entry

SUNDAY: It has been a very wet day which rather suited my dizzy mood. I've been a bit clumsy and stressed. Not able to focus on anything and at lunch time I lost control of my soup bowl which flew across the table and shattered on the floor. Wet shards and tears everywhere. Ash, bless him, didn't say anything just helped me tidy up. Later, he was trying to talk to me while I was making tea but I was completely unable to do two things at once. So, another wobble & collapse. It isn't fair that he ends up dealing with the remains of the day. Feeling low and anxious so think it is time to register it as a migraine. Am a bit apprehensive about going to the office tomorrow. Not sure exactly why I'm so scared. Perhaps because I'm going back to something I know hasn't been good for me lately? Bed soon I think and I'll have to take a view tomorrow over work.

I cancelled all my social activities and did nothing but work, sleep and eat for two weeks. It worked; in that I was able to do all my work hours that fortnight. One evening, while walking back from the bus stop after a frustrating day in the office, I realised I wasn't happy anymore. That I'd lost that lovely feeling of contentment which I had at Christmas. Sometime in the last few months of clinics and work and trying to build a life, I'd lost my Perspective. The evening sunshine was warm, kids ran past smiling but I felt stretched and fragile. *Tissue thin. Again. Things need to change. Again.*

Chapter 14

Fatigue management in the wild

Harder, faster, stronger

June: Two years and three months after the incident

Summer started with a phone call to the boss. 'Morning Alder, do you have a minute please?'

'Of course, it's good timing. But this doesn't sound good?'

'No, I'm... Well, I'm struggling again.'

'I was wondering. Your current use of annual leave isn't sustainable. Is it all going on migraines?'

'Yes. Lots of little ones or one big one, we don't know.'

'What did the dizzy docs say?'

'Do better and keep going, basically.'

'Hmm.'

'The "graduated return" says I should be full time by now, but four days a week is too much. So, I'd like to drop back to three days again for the next fortnight.'

'Well, to make things easier, why don't we try three days a week for all of June?'

'The whole month? Would that work for the team?'

'It's about what works for you. And going by the calendar month will make it easier for the rest of the department to remember.'

'Yes, that makes sense. Thank you, I'm sorry about this.'

'Not at all, we just want you back to normal. It doesn't matter how long it takes.'

As he spoke, he must have been thinking of the discussions needed to sort out the change. Asking managers to ensure cover in the department, letting HR and the payroll team know... I didn't think about that until later, until it was too late to thank him properly. All I felt at the time was relief.

Email to parents

ME: I'm now only working Mondays, Wednesdays and Fridays so that I get a full day of rest after each day in the office. Am really pleased with the change even though it has only been two weeks! Network connection problems on Monday led to moving desks three times. I ended up working in an open plan office with the whole department for the first time. The noise had been anticipated, and I was armed with my headphones and timers to ensure breaks.

Something I hadn't foreseen was that sitting closer to my team meant working on their deadlines, not mine. As well as working to other people's expectations, an additional stress was being pulled into meetings, too. It was a relief to cycle home at the end of the day and know it would be a full day before I had to be back. I do love being able to cycle-commute again, the ride helps me to leave much of the stress behind.

In the days off I've done nothing but rest, though I did get to do both tai chi and yoga for the first time in ages. I haven't been doing them often recently and my balance & clumsiness have become noticeably worse. Nice to know they work when I do them! So, have rewritten the Fatigue Management Planner again to fit them in and work out of this dizzy spell.

I'm also able to pay attention to the garden after a long absence. My inner-city wildlife mini-pond has only been in four months and already damsel flies are laying eggs. Success! Hoping to pimp my pond out to dragon flies next. Oh, the rock and roll life I lead.

July: Two years and four months after the incident

Diary entries

MONDAY: Ugh, the weekend was another write-off. Despite my optimism last month, I'm still finding work hard. Another migraine today and another day of annual leave.

WEDNESDAY: Even with four days away from the office I was anxious last night. Am worrying about doing the right thing now that I don't have the vocational rehabilitation or vestibular physiotherapy teams to guide me. Can't believe the dizzy doc appointments are six months apart! It makes for a long wait full of uncertainty. But this morning I felt up to the office and colleagues again. Seems they were a bit worried about me, don't blame them. Alder asked for a meeting first thing.

'Grab a seat. Is that rosemary tea?'

The dried herb swirled round the mug in my hand. 'Yeah, coffee is still off limits as a possible migraine trigger. And they say rosemary helps with memory.'

'Is that an official prescription?'

'No, but I'm willing to try anything that won't cause harm.'

'Are things still a struggle? We were worried about Monday.'

'From what I can tell, the migraine was caused by a morning in bright sunlight. But don't really know.'

'Is that all it takes?'

'Not usually, but I'm still catching up on myself after going back to three days a week. It seems to be working though.'

'I'm glad it is working. I think we need to formalise your return. You've effectively been on pay-as-you-go and using up time in lieu, annual leave or sick leave for over two years now.'

'I can't believe it has been so long.'

'It has, but then your injury was serious.'

'It's been a long road, I forget that sometimes.'

'Speaking of a long road, I have news. It's finally time I retired again. For good this time.'

'Oh! Right, well…'

'Is that too much of a shock?'

'No, no. I knew it was coming. When you took the job, you said it would only be for five years. It's just, I forget how much time I lost sometimes.'

'Say that after a 40-year career.'

'Yeah, wow. When will you go? You'll be missed.'

'Not for a while. It's hush–hush at the moment as there are some things to sort out first.'

'That sounds ominous.'

'It should, you are one of those "things". To take a leaf out of the vocational rehabilitation team's play book, I'd like to consolidate you on a three day per week fixed term contract. We can have an option of adding more days as and when you are ready.'

'Ok… that makes sense.'

'You don't have to agree now, talk with your husband and sleep on it. It would just give all of us, you and the team, some clarity.'

'I can let you know when I'm in again.'

'Take your time and tell me next week. I'd just like to make sure your position is sorted before the next director comes along.'

'The "next director". You know, I used to think that would be me. How times change.'

Alder cleared his throat. 'The team are saying it is nice to have you back. It hasn't been the same in the office without you.'

'It really is good to be back working with people again. It's just louder and busier than I'd expected.'

'You know you can still take breaks whenever you need.'

'I do, it's just sometimes hard to tell when I need one.'

'Do the doctors know if that is normal?'

'Apparently some people with brain injury tend to lack insight. I might be one of them, but then, how would I know?'

It took me a while to work out why he was laughing.

Diary entries

WEDNESDAY: A bit woozy this morning so decided against the cycle commute. It was a wrench as the weather was beautiful, but a dizzy head said that I'd better take the train and be safe. Walked to the local station only to find it was closed, which wasn't announced online. Ah, public transport – the great disrupter of Fatigue Management Planners! So, I resigned myself to being late for the morning meeting. I've noticed that if I just accept things my anxiety drops as I avoid the thoughts of 'if I do this, or if only I'd done that.' On to the bus instead and managed to make the necessary changes to the Fatigue Management Planner. That new plan went straight out the window too. I was late for the first meeting, as predicted. But once that was over, I was asked into two more 'emergency' meetings. At the manager's request my project was put on hold and I ended up spending the day helping others out. I was going to stay late to make up for the problems in the morning. But half an hour catching up turned into two hours as a colleague wanted to discuss her plans following Alder's resignation. Interesting, and I'm glad my advice is still valued. But I finally left at 7pm with a cracking headache and still very tired now. Panadol and an early bed tonight.

FRIDAY: Today was supposed to be a day in the office but I woke before the alarm and knew it wouldn't be. It has been a fiercely hot couple of days, with the temperature getting up to 33 yesterday. I've been worried about how my migraines and fatigue would cope in the heat – I'm already drinking gallons of water to try and stay cool. My headache seems to have been building with the heat and this morning I was struggling to stand and talk again. It was a bit cooler today, but the damage had already been done and I used up more annual leave. I did manage to sleep through a lot of the dizziness which is a relief.

THURSDAY: End of the month already and I will be going back on contract. Or at least I emailed Alder and agreed to his suggestion. I didn't see him at work today, but was glad of a quiet day as I did make it to social activity! A catch up in a pub and saw my friends for the first time in weeks. I'd had to move my work days round to ensure I would have Friday to rest, but it was worth it. I was thrilled to see everyone on what proved to be a long but successful night. Perry said I seem to be getting back to normal again which was really nice to hear. Proof that I am getting there. Really pleased that this week I managed three days' work, to commute by bike and even see friends. Hurray for progress!

August: Two years and five months after the incident

Diary entry

SUNDAY: I've not completed the diary since Wednesday evening. What a failure! But then, it shows that I really have been struggling the last few days. I've been having trippy dreams and spent a good deal of time spacing out again. I'd switched my days to try and rest before Perry's birthday on the weekend so was in the office on Thursday and off on Friday for a change. Thursday was busy at work; nothing had really changed. There were still big problems with the website and audit plans so the manager said that my project can taking a leaping jump for the moment. It made sense for her but no one has told the CEO. He has been telling customers I'll sort things out for them and not remembering I only work part time. With all that, I forgot to set my alarm and take breaks. I find it hard to rest when working with other people. In good news, Alder let me know that he has confirmed my three day per week contract. A massive relief as am barely managing again. Glad they aren't expecting me to work full time in the near future.

Friday was pretty much a write off, I had very trippy dreams and felt very woozy on waking. My day off was filled with dozing. I didn't feel up to doing anything productive and ignored everything. Saturday was supposed to be a beer festival for Perry's birthday. I was still exhausted, so husband headed off alone. Again. Found myself just sitting in the garden zoning out for most of the time. Sunday has proven an odd mix, still really tired and have once more am frustrated with the 'tired of being tired' feeling. Plus, I'm annoyed that the spike in stress at work seems to have taken me days to deal with.

Email to self

- Tell manager that I still need to have one day a week working from home.
- Sort website issues.
- Email other department re: delay to their new project request.
- Sort hours for HR for next few weeks.
- Chase insurance case again.

Audit day at the office

Alder and the managers had been focused on this day for weeks. My experience with past inspections meant I had been drafted in too. All my projects had been put on hold and I'd been fending off queries from other departments about them. I wasn't involved on the day, but hours of my work had gone into the reports and on helping others prepare their teams for any queries. After a tense morning, Alder walked the auditor from the building. It was an open plan office; everyone could see that **a decision** had been made. All eyes were on the door when Alder returned. 'We passed!'

Cheers and whoops mingled with cries of 'Mine's a pint!'

'Congratulations everyone, well done. While it was of course a team effort, I'd like to give special thanks to several people…'

Huh, not me. Guess I was only on the periphery to them. But it took up all my hours for weeks.

Another manager interrupted these thoughts. 'I'd also like to give a special mention to those who have worked on a different project. The website update has been a long and fraught task over many months.'

Yes, it took me ages to design and build the customer interface. Thank goodness I managed to finish it before you needed me for the audit.

'It hasn't been easy but it is a fantastic new upgrade which simply wouldn't be working without the efforts of…'

Ignored again? But I pointed out all the issues which you said weren't a problem and then tried to find solutions when they bit you in the…

As the department faded back to work, I made excuses and went for a much-needed break. Indignation had given way to puzzlement. The entire department had no idea of the work I'd done in the last year. *I guess it is because I've been in that separate office most of the time.* It was illuminating. *You mean infuriating!*

A cup of tea in the sun helped to rearrange my perspective. I came to see this as a timely prompt to ensure it didn't happen again, especially with a new director imminent. The rest of the morning was spent writing up all the projects I'd worked on in the last year to inform the newcomer of my work. And I chased the insurance case. Again.

Diary entry

FRIDAY: End of another week, nearly the end of another month but definitely the end of Alder's career. He had only been with the company for seven or eight years but had had quite an influence. Initially, he was a liaison in another department and we had become firm friends. With a depth of experience behind him, he was quickly promoted to director of my department, and my direct boss. We had managed that for a year, it can be a delicate balance when you end up at a party with your boss on a Friday evening, but we had coped. After the incident, he was a strong support both in the office and as a friend. Now he is gone. It's only afterwards that you realise how much someone has done for you. I'll probably never know how much work he had put in to manage my team and to keep HR off my back. But he had a good send off at least. Once the usual company speeches were done our entire department decamped to a beer garden and the party started. Alder and I managed to speak to each other early on, we both know I still can't manage in parties for long. When I left about eight, they were getting seriously settled in. Oh, to have been there!

September: Two years and six months after the incident

Tweet

Two years ago, our new woman's football team was a daydream, now it's about to enter a competitive league. Awesome job by the committee!

Email to Hazel

ME: Not much to report here, awful migraines during that wee heatwave so am glad summer has returned to normal. On a three day per week contract, trying to meet friends, hoping to get to a footy training … not much has changed really. This email won't be a long one as the Planner says I need to fit in my yoga again. Man, my balance has deteriorated!

Diary entry

FRIDAY: Just been reading back through my diaries. It helps to see just how much things have progressed. Especially after a slow day like today. Work was, well, I'm going to write about it less in the hope that my anxiety over it drops too. Anxiety is definitely my kryptonite now – just writing this bit about how anxiety affects me is making me anxious. I will get a handle on it – hey I've come this far. But it is still frustrating. I have been reading up on fatigue and the migraines. Migraine diary shows that most migraines start in the morning. So, decided to move the trippy pills to 7.30 now as that is exactly 12 hours before I need to be up most mornings. If I'm already pushing it to wake up with the last effects of the pills that might be a factor in how often I'm getting migraines? It feels odd to be making things up as I go, but so much of the advice from the experts in this recovery is 'suck it and see.' I'm getting the hang of my Fatigue Management Planner again and am finding time for the 'anti-dizzy' exercises like yoga, cycling and tai chi. I do think it has helped as I'm feeling pretty good tonight, tired but not wiped out, despite doing quite a lot and waking with a thick head yesterday, progress!

Tweet

Teacher: 'You need to work on your "falling leaf hands" before we get into "wave hands like clouds".' Sometimes tai chi is exactly what you expect…

October: Two years and seven months after the incident

Diary entry

MONDAY: Damn it, I'm really frustrated today. Friday was an office day but I managed it well. I took all my breaks, declined the invitation to a pub lunch and made sure it was an easy day. I followed that up with a quiet Saturday, of gentle exercise and taking things carefully. It was all to get ready for a Sunday afternoon with Rose. She is over from the United States for the first time in years. Despite the many people who want to see her, she had cleared Sunday afternoon for a quiet catch up, just the two of us. We had a lovely, if short, three hours in a park with a carefully monitored two units of alcohol. It was a far cry from how we used to party together but it was so good to see her! An awesome afternoon and I felt normal again. But today is a write off. Dizziness, headaches, trouble walking…gah! What do I have to do to get better?

Tweet

First experiment with alcohol since a brain injury two years ago was not successful. Back to being teetotal and to finding creative uses for the wine judging glasses. Behold, a flower vase!

Diary entry

FRIDAY: Migraine? Certainly, I woke feeling decidedly woozy, I remember thinking in bed that I shouldn't push my health for the sake of work. But when so much of my willpower is used up on just moving, I fall back into the pattern of pushing through. By the end of the day I was rather pissed off with myself at having gone in to work. Poor husband got it in the evening – really not the end to the day that we would want. At least Ash is happy in his new job. The pay means we could manage on his salary alone. That thought is a massive bonus in my recovery and as the insurance case drags on.

November: Two years and eight months after the incident

Diary entry

TUESDAY: Autumn has turned today and it has been cold, grey, dull and drizzly. Winter is definitely just around the corner and I had a big sleep in to celebrate. That, combined with my fatigue today, has led me to believe that I still need more than nine hours sleep per night. Plus, I'm not really doing much with the extra time if I'm honest. The intent to do more reading is there, but by the time I get to it I'm so tired that nothing goes in. Back to the 10.30 bed times and to re-do the Fatigue Management Planner again.

Tweet

Played the cello loudly tonight: 'So kids in the flat upstairs, I see your ukulele & tambourine and raise you 20 years of bad practice!'

Diary entry

THURSDAY: Catching up on yesterday again. I just don't seem the have the energy or will to do the diary on evenings when I have been in the office. I had a cracking headache last night and it seems to have hung around today too. Yesterday was a long day in the office. I did use the timers more often but still getting the 'shafts of anxiety' and not seeing the bigger picture. It didn't help that another emergency meeting led to another priority project landing in my lap. That rather set the tone of an unstructured day. In the end I went out for walk and returned with a packet of skittles and some chocolate. Throw in a bowl of cereal and you get a working lunch. I can just hear the dizzy docs 'that isn't a balanced diet, you need to watch sugar spikes as they can bring on migraines.' Yeah, I know. But we can't be a saint every day. Wrote up most of the project that afternoon, but decided to sit on it until my next office day. I want to be helpful but not give the impression that I have nothing else to do. Ah, work is frustrating. I'm getting there and do need to keep reminding myself of that. Today I moved the pills back to 8pm after my trial of having them at 7.30pm. I have been waking earlier in the morning, which seems pointless now that the sun isn't up, and getting brain fog earlier in the evening. I am not on the bicycle until after 8.30am so that ensures I'm not cycling within twelve hours of taking the pills. The change will mean taking the pills surreptitiously in the middle of yoga class. It shouldn't affect my balance for a few hours but... another thing to monitor, I guess.

December: Two years and nine months after the incident

Diary entry

WEDNESDAY: The most interesting thing that happened today happened on the ride into the office. A car passed me and drove up to a red light, using up most of the designated cyclist-only box despite having plenty of time to stop earlier. When myself and the other cyclists packed into the small cycling space left in front of his car, the driver went berserk. Sounding his horn, shouting abuse… It was scary but stupid. I tried to laugh because really, what else can you do? There was a cycle courier in the bunch and I asked him how he deals with road rage. He replied 'I've been doing this twenty years, so have seen everything. You aren't going to change anyone's perspective in a minute waiting at the lights. Eventually you run out of things to say.' For some reason it really struck me, he relies on cycling for his job but had a 'let it go' attitude which shields him from anxiety over other's actions. Can I get that too? Another busy day getting my head down to try to meet the project deadline. Worked till nearly six and suddenly it is 10pm.

Email reminder to self

ME: Dig out last email re: work insurance case and resend to HR as another request for them to sort it out.

Diary entry

NEW YEAR'S EVE 2016: Well, in another return to normality I've joined those ranks of people who get sick at Christmas. It is an 'Improvement' I could have done without to be honest. But it did flag up another 'Improvement' which I might have missed. The fog caused by the cold meant the days have melted easily into one another. I sat down to fill in this diary and found that I'd missed a day, that I couldn't remember Friday at all. Even after Ash confirmed the date, I still had trouble believing that I'd lost a day. But this time I know it isn't the brain injury. I didn't even think that it might be. Once I would automatically attribute all my lapses and forgetfulness to the brain injury. Now I'm finding the real culprits, in this case a cold, without assuming it could be my fault. Chuffed with that change of Perspective so had more chocolate to celebrate. Sadly, I won't be celebrating when the fireworks go off. This cold means there will be another new year brought in in bed.

2017 and 2018: Pacing

Chapter 15

Into the third year of recovery
Wait, is this normal?

January: Two years and ten months after the incident

Summary of reply from local brain injury charity

COORDINATOR: Thank you for your interest in the new writing class. I have signed you up and Hawthorn, the teacher, will expect you at the end of the month.

Diary entry

WEDNESDAY: Back to work for the new year. Cycled to work to learn that my bike lock & other belongings had been thrown out over Christmas. The facilities manager had merrily binned the lot despite them being carefully stored in a named box with a note saying 'Please don't throw out, call xxxxxxxxxx if any problems'. I asked him if that meant the company would reimburse me for the losses. Suspect his answer of 'asking HR about it' meant it was being kicked into the long grass along with my insurance claim. Two things to chase them about now.

Email to parents

ME: Not much else to report here, work is busy gearing up for its 'event of the year' which sadly I have a huge amount to do with. I've been working on days off as work has been frantic. The big day is Monday and am trying to organise a third of it while being ignored by the department I'm supposedly helping. But a colleague in a completely unrelated department who has never had anything to do with the event took the time to critique my work. Seriously, what is it that makes a man feel the need to tell me exactly how to do my job despite the fact they have never done it and have little idea on how it works? Sigh, such a shame as we used to get on well but working with him is now a nightmare. Generally feeling fed up with work. Every year this part of the event is a full-time job, now I'm trying to do it three days a week so have been working quite late. Even the janitor has been asking me to leave so that he can lock up. Ash has been on the receiving end of my frustration and stress. The sheer fatigue of trying to keep up has led to another three-day dizzy migraine which I've just had to work through.

Diary entry

MONDAY: Today was the main event I've been working so hard for. I was in bed early on last night as anticipated a long day today. However, problems started overnight as I woke with a terrible thirst but didn't realise my leg muscles were paralysed. I made it upright but promptly fell over and bounced off the wardrobe. Ash was startled awake with the noise which he thought was an earthquake. I was trying to reassure him while dealing with the odd sensation of not being able to move my leg at all. Was this paralysis some odd effect of these trippy pills? It has only happened the one time, that I know of. Perhaps my muscles often turned off in my sleep, I wouldn't know. Eventually my leg woke up and we got me off the floor and back to bed. Found out in the morning that I'd pulled the muscles while trying to get them back into life. So, I was hobbling through a whirlwind day and our flagship event. Thankfully everyone was also too busy to notice. The day was a blur of trying to sort out last minute problems while others alternately gave me orders before saying it was up to me and then blaming me for things that were not my fault. But the important thing is that the clients were happy and rewarded. That was the aim of my last six months of work so will pat myself on the back.

'Yes, you need a break. But don't expect to want one.' The words of my vocational rehabilitation therapist come back to tease me, too late to prevent the migraine.

The tinnitus echoes, constantly ringing against the steady beat of the headache. Pain throbbing behind the eyes as the teeth grit to force me onwards. Throwing everything I have into the fight. Fighting to get better, but failing and falling back into the sticky treacle of fatigue.

I must get better, I will get better, I am getting better. The will to fight, to prove that I will not stop here. I will not admit defeat and live the half-life I'm terrified of falling into. I must get better, I will get better, I am better.

Then why do I feel this way? Why am I home, watching the drizzle create patterns in the puddles on a dull dreary afternoon? If I'm better, why am I still here?

The sparkles whir in my view, the precursor to another migraine. The ethereal proof, visible only to myself, that I have once again failed, have pushed things too far and will inevitably fall again into the dark silence of another day of half-life. While others carry on. If I'm better, why am I still here?

The computer sways, the desk seems to flow, fluid under my hands. The world that seemed so certain and solid is insubstantial, in motion. Time to give up again, time to resign myself to hours of quiet, trying to stay still while the world swims taunting the pain in my head. To get better, I must be still, here.

Do I think too much about myself? Wrapped up in this pain and whirling it is easy to forget. There are people out there, people worth getting better for. It is time to be still. To be here.

Diary entry

FRIDAY: Catching up on my diary entries again. Not much to report beyond another three days of migraines this week. Two weeks on and I'm still trying to recover from the frantic rush of my employer's event. I have missed days of work and several planned events with friends. The view from bed is dull now that the tree has been cut down.

February: Two years and eleven months after the incident

Clinic notes: Neuro-otology/dizzy docs

I reviewed the patient today and was pleased to hear that, despite recent problems, her extensive migraine tracker shows that headache and vestibular symptoms have improved since the middle of last year. She now presents with approximately two to three migraine headaches per month. These have 'milder' vestibular symptoms consisting of a feeling of unsteadiness and a sensation of movement. The patient has also reduced her working hours and is now working three days per week which has made a difference with regards to her level of stress. We discussed presentation of migraine symptoms and management in clinic today. The patient is doing general exercises which involve balance such as yoga and cycling. She has noted a benefit with regard to her balance and I have encouraged her to continue with these. She is at present taking amitriptyline 60mg per day. Depending on her level of symptoms the amitriptyline could be further increased as required, by 10mg per fortnight, up to maximum of 150mg per day. However, should symptoms improve, I also discussed with the patient that she could try to gradually reduce the amitriptyline, again reducing by 10mg every week or every other week. I have arranged for the patient to be reviewed in clinic in six months' time.

The dizzy doctor was surprised and thrilled to see a patient with such a detailed spreadsheet tracking migraines over a full year. As well as noting the onset and length of migraines, my migraine diary also recorded where the migraine started, what the auras were, any missed activities, all the symptoms and possible triggers.

In return, I was pleased to hear that the trippy pills might be able to help further. But again, the recovery instructions were to 'try it and see.' Increasing the pills might help to reduce my migraines, or it might just increase the side effects which also included dizziness and fatigue… Hmm.

Tweet

Have now cycled London in:

- sunshine
- frost/ice
- fog
- gales
- rain
- hail
- sleet
- strikes/protests
- riots
- Olympics
- with police escort
- and FINALLY, snow!

March: Three years after the incident

Diary entry

THURSDAY: Another anniversary arrives and this one has brought with it the realisation that I need to get some structure back again. Had a very dizzy and painful head this morning so treated myself to a sleep in. It was a gorgeous day so I chose to walk to writing class and get the exercise in that way. Class started slowly, I guess mine wasn't the only brain injury playing up. In the end, class was productive though I felt a little flighty and dizzy throughout, I hope that didn't show. Our teacher, Hawthorn, has suggested that, now that the three of us have a handle on the basics, we write a story together. Admit I was cautious of mingling the frustrations of three people who are struggling with fatigue, attention or memory problems in an attempt to co-operate. But she must know what she is doing and it will teach me patience!

Tweet

Yay! Three weeks migraine free :)

Seems I'm celebrating by having a migraine :(

Last diary entry

SUNDAY: I just sat down to do another epic catch up of missed diary entries and realised that I'm seeing this diary more as a chore than anything else. It isn't really happening and I just get spikes of guilt when I do remember it. As my recovery has gone on, some things have dropped away, like tai chi, to be replaced with others; I feel more inspired by yoga at the moment. Perhaps it is time to put the diary to one side for a while to concentrate on other things. The alarm reminders on my phone have been decimated and I've pared the Fatigue Management Planner right back to the basics. For the next wee while I'll do things for enjoyment rather than because I have to. Let's see how that goes. Perhaps I'll even get in some planned spontaneity :)

April: Three years and one month after the incident

> **Tweet**
> Walking alone along a residential street in broad daylight and was harassed and had my arm 'stroked' by creepy man – in 2017!?

It really is just as it sounds. I was walking home from another GP appointment in the early evening. An unseasonably hot afternoon had emptied the streets as people baked in the local parks. A door opened on the other side of the road and a man came out. He saw me and crossed over while calling out: 'Hey.'

'Afternoon.'

'Hey, want some fun?'

'No.' I gripped my bag closer.

'But you shouldn't be alone on a gorgeous afternoon.' He was walking next to me now, keeping pace as I sped up.

'I'm going home to my husband.' *Emphasise the husband bit. Someone knows where I am and is expecting me.*

'I'm sure he won't mind. I need company.' He reached out and stroked my arm.

'Go away and leave me alone.'

'No need to be like that.' He grabbed at my elbow.

I twisted out of his grip and sped up. 'F*ck off, leave me alone.'

'You f*cking b*tch.'

Why do some men just assume women owe them?

May: Three years and two months after the incident

Summary of email from Hawthorn, the writing teacher

ME: Hi class, attached is my edit of the main part of our story. What I would like a.s.a.p from each of you is a last paragraph or sentence. We might end up with three different endings. It is coming on so well, almost to perfection.

Summary of emails with parents

ME: Yesterday at work I felt like I was continually pushing and wasn't letting myself relax, indeed due to the headache I didn't get to bed till after 11. Most of the morning was a meeting during which I was fantasising about how relaxing it would be if I was fired. I wouldn't feel this tired and stressed all the time. The meeting started over an hour late, lasted for ages and we learnt nothing new, made no decisions nor got anything done. Instead it followed the predictable interdepartmental format of 'gripe by email but everything is fine face to face'. Three hours written off. I know that is standard for business meetings but I'd never noticed before. The brother had told me that after his brain injury he lost patience with the minutiae of daily life, perhaps I've done the same?

Finally managed to get into my email inbox only discover that the client couldn't use our conference call software. Rather than deal with it yesterday, my colleagues had passed the problem on to me despite it being my day off. This meant I now needed to select and install a new programme before the conference call in an hour's time. I didn't want to randomly download software to the company servers so contacted the company Helpdesk who were their usual brilliant help: 'We know nothing and seriously can't you give us a bit of warning?' I really wanted to reply with 'Well, no. I only work three days a week and was stuck in a meeting all morning. The remote desktop problems you haven't solved over the past weeks meant I couldn't access my emails until now. I don't know why our colleagues chose to pass the problem on to me instead of contacting you yesterday. However, you've had just as much warning as me only this is your job.'

Blah, getting frustrated just thinking about it. Anyway, I remembered my CBT lessons: remove your feelings from it and find a solution. So, the actual reply read: 'Sorry guys, first I've heard of this too. Ok, I'll sort it myself.' Still getting spikes of anxiety, but managing to react better to them.

MUM: Yes, company meetings are always like that, we just need to grin and bear them. Or claim you need a cognitive break and leave? As to the computer problems, you were taking on too much there. Colleagues chose to dump on you because they didn't want to deal with the Helpdesk. The Helpdesk haven't solved your connection problems because you take it upon yourself to work around the difficulties despite the strain that places on you. This wasn't a case of your brain injury slowing you down, this was a case of other people taking advantage. Not a criticism, but just take a breath next time and maybe stop doing other people's jobs for them.

Tweet

Turn on my newly assigned office computer and Windows is running update 200 out of 21,478 – this is not going to be a productive day…

June: Three years and three months after the incident

Email to friends

ME: Hope you all survived the heatwave, we didn't move to London for this kind of weather! My migraines don't do well in the heat but I can read again without a headache so am calling that a 'win!' Next week looks a bit cooler so perhaps time for an evening tipple? I've found a central pub with a craft beer festival which is doggy friendly. All hail my search algorithms.

'Mine's a half.'

'I don't buy halfs'

'Well, the brain injury means I've not really drunk alcohol for over three years and I'm on these amazing mind-bending pills so…'

Perry grinned. 'Turns out, I do buy halfs. But only for you.'

It was an awesome evening of fun and laughter. I felt ok after half a pint so had one more then stuck to water to wash down the pill at 8pm. The next two hours flew by and then I turned into a zombie. It was obvious even to the slightly drunken Perry: 'Are you ok? You look zoned out a bit.'

'It's the pills, I just felt them start to work. It must be nearly 10.'

'On the dot. Wow, that really is like clockwork.'

'Yeah, time for me to head off early again. What a pain!'

'Hey, you lasted much longer than last time. It is so nice to see you getting back to normal again.'

'One day I'll be back matching you pint for pint.'

'I dare you!'

Tucked into a seat on the bus home I grinned stupidly at the darkened city streets rolling past. *That was a great evening, I stayed out for ages.* Unlike my attempts at socialising over the past two years, I hadn't spent the evening in a dizzy haze of pain. My hands no longer gripped the table to stay still as I fought off the encroaching fatigue. Trying to stay in the happy moments, to cling to my friends and their company for a few more moments before time came. That inevitable time when had to go, to miss out again. *But you were there longer tonight.* I used to stay for an hour or two. Tonight, I'd been part of the fun for nearly five hours before the trippy fog descended again. *Nearly back to normal then?*

The next morning was a nightmare. And not just because of the horrid trippy dreams, though there were there again too. More of those 'there's someone in the house but you are completely unable to do anything' dreams which are always freaky and disturbing. But this time there was an added terror. *Oh, sh*t, I'm dizzy. Not again! Oh, I hate this.* Ash got up and tucked me in again. 'But, I only had a pint…'

I felt awful, spinning in space again. Long forgotten shafts of pain worked into the arm muscles again as I gripped the bed and tried not to cry. *I said I never wanted to feel like this again. I've failed again.*

July: Three years and four months after the incident

'So, booze. Not a huge success then?'

'No, I felt awful and tired and such a…' I couldn't speak around the lump in my throat. Tears rolled down cheeks and I struggled not to cry. *Not in public!*

Laurel dropped her salad on the park bench and dragged me in for a quick hug. 'What the…? Where did that come from?'

I managed a shaky breath. 'Sorry, sorry. I'm fine now.'

We turned back to our salads and Laurel ate in silence for a time. All my friends had become adept at this now. At giving me a quiet moment to collect my thoughts.

'Sorry, it is really good to see you after so long. That was just… well. I'm just tired and deeply disappointed in myself.'

'Disappointed? But look how far you've come. You are so much better than three months ago, let alone three years.'

'I know it's just…'

'What? Spit it out.'

'I had one pint, and left early, yet still had a migraine which wrote an entire day off! I just really want to be normal again. And all these men keep attacking or think they know better than me. And work is an absolute nightmare. People give me tasks and then constantly prevent me from doing them by giving me other ones before interrupting me again to ask me why I haven't done the first project yet. It's all just…'

'Normal.'

I was stunned by her interruption. 'What?'

Laurel was smirking at me. 'Usually when we have lunch you are talking about fitting in a ton of hospital appointments, not being able to sleep thanks to trippy pills, being too dizzy to walk but having to do weird exercises with cushions while waiting on the results of your last scan.'

'I still have the pills. Think I'm getting used to them. But everything else is…'

'Normal. It's all just normal. Work is pissing you off. Men are trying to push you around and make you do what they want. And you went to a pub then had a hangover. Congratulations. You are back to normal.'

I stared at her. *What the hell?*

'Are you ok? Have you zoned out again?'

'No, I'm just thinking… Are you serious?'

'You are so busy trying to fight off the same things as everyone else that you haven't noticed what you aren't dealing with any more. You are getting busy again and have been so desperate to get back to normal that you haven't noticed how close you are.'

'Huh.'

Laurel triumphantly devoured the last of her salad, and I watched the world go by.

'You mean, I'm spending all this time complaining about regular stuff.'

'Exactly. Like normal people do.'

Chapter 16

Brain injury survivor
Who am I now?

All those months fighting to be normal, to grump conspiringly at the office water cooler, to sit with my friends on a Friday evening, to walk down a street without fear. Three years into the recovery, I had achieved all those aims and more, albeit with varying success. There were still relapses, times when I would have a cognitive lapse or just zone out and think of nothing for a few hours.

My friends and family had helped me to rebuild this normality, and pointed out when I achieved it. Life hadn't bounced back to the way things were. I had expected that and had worked through the grief of lost opportunities and futures with counselling and therapy. But now that I had achieved my aims, I still wasn't quite happy with this new normal. I began to see that parts of me had changed too.

August: Three years and five months after the incident

Email to Laurel

ME: No, I'm not having the freaky dreams at the moment. Thank you for reminding me. It's good to have those prompts to show just how far I've come. I've even managed to fit in a day at the office and a party! Friday was Ash's office summer party and plus-ones were invited along. No booze for me, I'm wary of mixing alcohol and the trippy pills after last time. It was a lovely evening, though I'm not sure how conversation turned to the topic of my brain injury. And I'm still not sure how I feel about sharing it with complete strangers. But come up it did and now I'm worried. I fear that they will judge me. I think that is what is making me unhappy now. I worry about how people will view me now that I am someone with a brain injury, a 'brain injury survivor.'

I had come across that term several times by now. It was used by the charity I had contacted for advice and was widely used online and in social media. People would describe themselves as a 'brain injury survivor' or as caring for a 'brain injury survivor.' It was a new concept, this idea of defining someone by their impediment. It was in summer that I was first asked: 'And are you a brain injury survivor?'

I hesitated. *Is that who I am now?* The woman took my pause for shyness and her smile broadened. 'You are welcome, everyone here understands what it is like.'

'Here' was my local branch of the brain injury charity, though the venue was still an hour away by public transport. The distance meant that I had been unable to fit their monthly meeting into the Fatigue Management Planner until now. The members included brain injury survivors and their families, as well as medical professionals and lawyers who were volunteering with the charity. It was reassuring to speak with those who could relate over the struggle with pathological fatigue or share strategies to cope with cognitive lapses.

It turned out that many families had received the 'you have a small window of healing' advice too. I'd read it was six months, others heard it was a year, still others were told 'a few years.'

'It's not true.' Dark eye's flashed and a withered hand struck the top of a walking cane. The man's speech had been blurred ever since an ABI years previously. Beside him, his wife and carer nodded firmly and took up the tale.

'We were told that, and I despaired. Oh, how I worried! A year came and went and he still needed a wheelchair. Two years later he started harder physiotherapy, and didn't he moan about it?!'

Her husband chuckled and they shared a smile before she continued. 'For his birthday that year, I bought him a cane. I said "You'll use that soon. You will be out of the chair before your next birthday." And he was.'

The man pointed at the cane resting on the back of his chair. 'Nearly three years after the injury, I walked down the street again. So, don't think about a "window of healing", just keep trying a little every day.'

It was also a sobering experience. I met victims of assault and traffic collisions as well as those who had an 'organic' brain injury, where a stroke or heart attack had been the cause. Most attendees had been hospitalised for many months and were still struggling with the effects years later. The fact that I was able to work caused a stir and an interrogation of 'how do you cope?' It was an interesting and exhausting evening.

The timing was serendipitous, my first visit to the local brain injury charity coincided with a national campaign to raise awareness about brain injuries in football. While I had donated to the charity after their helpful advice, this was my first chance to volunteer my time, to give something back. Of course, I couldn't do much in between the return to work and ongoing migraines but I was determined to participate.

In snatched moments on my days off I emailed the clubs, leagues and football associations whom I had worked with over the years. Almost everyone was happy to help raise awareness of such an important issue and asked for more information. Each reply or re-tweet brought a broad smile and a sense of purpose. I wanted more.

Summary of emails with local brain injury charity

CO-ORDINATOR: Thanks so much for asking about the communications volunteering role. I'll do my best to give you a full, detailed, description of what we do below so you can decide if there is something you'd like to help with. There are several channels of communication so of course you might want to think about helping with one or two that interest you.

ME: I'm happy to help with something for the next newsletter and it seems ideal to write about the writing class if that is ok? Tweet-wise, I've come across a few stories in connection with brain injury. Would you like me to email you links, or write complete tweets with mentions and hashtags so you can just re-tweet them?

September: Three years and six months after the incident

Tweet

Even after terrible incidents, pros with top medical care struggle to get brain injuries diagnosed & treated. Article → 'Rugby League: Lance Hohaia's nightmare head knocks.' By Michael Burgess.

Summary of emails with parents

ME: I spent the morning searching the web for brain injury stories which might be relevant to the volunteer work I'm doing. One of the news feeds turned up a report on a professional rugby league player and the problem he had with a brain injury. He had been attacked in an 'off the ball' incident and then punched again while lying unconscious on the pitch. It was a horrible incident, the game stopped immediately and the team doc was with him within seconds. The problems he had getting his brain injury recognised and treated despite having top level medical care from the first minute made me realise that there wasn't anything different that might have happened with my injury. Even if I had been knocked out and hospitalised on the day, I could have easily had these problems. Sobering thought.

DAD: I was ruminating on your email while watching a rugby match here in New Zealand. One of the captains was knocked out cold. During the pause for medical attention, the band struck up to entertain the crowd while the commentators filled the time with 'hope you are keeping warm during the delay'. It struck me then. That people have become so used to seeing these kinds of injuries; that it's just a matter of distracting the crowd so they don't get irritated by the delay.

ME: Is it just that we are more aware of knocks to the head now? I do remember that in the pre-professional era players weren't lauded for stopping to give first aid to the opposition as they are now. It wasn't exceptional, rather stopping to help an injured player or give first aid was just the right thing to do. Now players are expected to ignore the damage done to a teammate, focus on only the game and carry on. It's horrible, and my experience with my former teammates shows the attitude is now being reflected at club level. Can we enjoy professional sports knowing how it contributes to terrible injuries?

October: Three years and seven months after the incident

Those thoughts were put into sharp perspective only a week or so later. I hadn't managed to spend much time with River FC over the summer. The team were several games into the new season before I was able to see them play.

It was a gorgeous autumn day, another perfect afternoon for football. In a hard-fought game River FC made a break and our striker, Fern, raced towards the opposition's penalty box. The final pass was just a little long and, despite a valiant chase, a defender got to the ball just before her. The centre-back thumped the ball hard, straight into Fern's hand.

Suddenly, Fern was screaming in pain and clutching at her wrist. The ref blew the whistle but no one else seemed to react. I grabbed the first aid kit and sprinted onto the pitch. Though I reached Fern quickly, it wasn't immediately clear what was wrong. She was clutching her arm and stag-gering around. 'Fern, what is it? Where is the pain?'

She just moaned and shook her head at me. *What do I do now?* Fern bounced from foot to foot but I helped her to sit down. Once Fern reached the ground, she curled over her hands. I sank down beside her and finally managed to see her right wrist. *Holy sh*t.* There were far too many lumps on her wrist and the thumb was at an odd angle. Her left hand was clamped around her right forearm, just above the lumps. There was so much pain that Fern was trying to control how much she had to feel. *Oh man, I've been there.*

It was obvious there was little to be done except get her to hospital. Another River FC supporter had joined me and, with careful encourage-ment, we helped Fern off the pitch. Her face was already alarmingly pale. As we walked slowly towards a nearby car, we could hear the game resume behind us. Though the journey through the city streets was quick, every bump in the road drew a soft, animal whimper from Fern. The driver dropped us off at the hospital and, once the A&E receptionist had signed us in, Fern and I were asked to take a seat and wait.

'What about painkillers?'

The receptionist paused at the sight of Fern's tight lips and white face. 'I'm sorry, I can't provide any. But the doctor will see her soon.'

Fern lowered herself gingerly onto the plastic chair and sat bolt upright. The pain was so intense that she hadn't spoken nor let go of her wrist since the injury. She was still rigid when pain relief showed up nearly an hour later. Eventually her name was called and we made our way into the depths of A&E. I knew it was a bad injury but an x-ray brought news which was worse than I'd imagined.

'Looks like the impact thrust the hand back, forcing the arm bone over the bone on the top of the wrist. There was also force sideways, creating problems at the base of the thumb, possibly a dislocation and break there too. Wow. You say this was a football?'

Fern just nodded. The nurse raised her eyebrow at me. 'Yeah, it was a centre-back clearance. Point blank range.'

'Unlucky. That's how I broke my wrist years ago too.'

'Umm, can she eat? We've not eaten for hours.'

'I'm sorry no. I think we'll need to manipulate the wrist back into posi-tion under sedation.'

What the hell does that mean? As a daughter of medics, I consider myself a veteran of A&E but I'd never heard that before. Suddenly I was no longer hungry and felt weak and light headed. *Get a grip, this isn't about you.* I hadn't thought it possible for Fern to turn paler, but I was wrong.

The nurse must have noticed too as she said it was time to get Fern onto a gurney. We followed her along another corridor and into a crowded room. *Uh oh! This is the emergency resuscitation room.* It was a really bad sign. Fern's injury was complicated enough that they had us in with heart attacks and traffic collisions. Fern was staring around wide-eyed, I pulled the curtain across to block the room from sight.

At length, four health workers filed into the tight space. After the introductions and explanations, it was down to business of 'manipulation under sedation'. Despite the phrase, Fern wasn't actually asleep. The medical team administered heavy-duty pain killers, but Fern was alert the whole time. I'll admit that the worst bit was the injections into the wrist, while I'm ok with needles, that depth and angle was a bit leg-shaking. Then four adults grunted and strained to manipulate Fern's wrist back into shape. The local anaesthetic meant Fern had no pain but she could still feel the bones move around. It looked awful and I have no idea how it must have felt.

After all that, I became fatigued and a dizzy fog descended. I didn't feel I could eat in front of Fern who still wasn't allowed food or water. Fern had said a few times that I could head off, that she'd be fine without me. I had been tempted but the look on her face when they'd said 'manipulation under sedation' convinced me to stay. *My mum would want someone to stay with me.*

At 10pm, after three more manipulations and hours after the injury, the A&E staff were at last happy with the position of Fern's wrist and set it in fast drying plaster. Before we could go, she was told to report the next day for an operation.

'An operation?' Fern's face was pale again and her good hand clutched for mine.

'Yes, the wrist is set ok for now. But we are concerned about the depth of the break into the joint.'

'It won't heal on its own?'

'It will but, well, we are worried about future use. This is a deep fracture in the wrist, if we leave it to heal on its own we suspect there will be limitations to future movement. An operation would reduce the risk but there will still likely be complications in later years, arthritis in particular.'

As the doctor spoke, I held Fern's hand tightly. *She is 23 and being told she will probably develop arthritis. At 23.* A few minutes later, I piled a dejected Fern into a black cab with a promise to text me as soon as she got home. I crawled onto a train, trying to ignore a nagging thought. *Never mind professional sports, can I even enjoy local football anymore?*

November: Three years and eight months after the incident

Summary of emails with Hazel

ME: I won't lie, I found the time in hospital with Fern exhausting, and sobering. Kept thinking about how similar a situation it had been to my injury, two players competing for the ball. As I showed at our last training session, I will never be able to join in a drill or kick-about without being competitive and so will always be at risk of another injury. Think you can see where my thoughts are going. I've decided it's time to step back from football and contact sports in general. That means giving up the Assistant Coach role. It has been a pleasure to help out and to get River FC off the ground. I'm sure there are great things to come!

HAZEL: Am gutted and you will be sorely missed. But I do understand where you're coming from. Before you disappear, I'd really appreciate one last bit of advice please. I have had an email from Fuchsia who has been out of the team for much of the summer with concussion. She wants to join again but hasn't been able to get a doctor's note to confirm she is fit to play. I'm not comfortable with this at all. We both know how serious concussion is!

ME: My two cents' worth would be to definitely stick to your guns and insist on a clearance to play. The risk is too high for the club. Head injuries differ from one to the other but that just makes it more difficult for doctors. To my mind, the most likely scenario would be that the GP doesn't feel comfortable giving Fuchsia a clearance to play. Even professional sports teams are still trying to work out how to deal with concussions. So, Fuchsia may not be able to get a simple yes or no from her doctor at all. Having said that, I think you are doing the right thing to protect her and the team. Stick to your guns!

It had been a long road, but my experience with brain injury was showing me how prevalent brain injury is, and it was also helping to shape the way people reacted to such injuries. Perhaps I could do more?

December: Three years and nine months after the incident

Summary of emails with neurology PhD researcher

ME: If you are still looking for lay members for your study steering committee, I would be interested in joining. I received an ABI which resulted in a brain bleed and vestibular migraines which were eventually treated through the NHS. I'm keen to give back so please let me know if you still need people.

RESEARCHER: Thanks for your email – yes, we are still looking for members! We have some government funded money to run a small trial investigating different treatments for dizziness following TBI. The purpose of the steering group is to ensure that when we write the protocol for the trial, we have input from a variety of people – including patients and/or career. This will help ensure the design and outcomes of the trial are relevant to patients and NHS services.

Email to psychology student at a research university

Please find attached the scanned survey on 'Coping Strategies following ABI' which you spoke about on Thursday at our brain injury writing group. I hope this file comes through ok, but do let me know if there are any problems.

Email to parents

The visit from the psychology student had been an interesting break from our writing collaboration exercises. Basically, it gave us a chance to help with data on how people recover after brain injury and what support could be put in place to help them. It led to interesting discussions of all our injuries. All our brain injuries are different, but they do have similarities. Despite my initial reservations, the other adult students and I have turned into decent companions fairly quickly. It is true that we are all bonded by our experiences, and our teacher's obvious enthusiasm has meant our creative output has grown exponentially. I'm exhausted after each class; it is like my brain has been busy filing through events or sorting out how I feel about things. Writing means that my creative side has had a bit more of a run out of late. As I write, my brain feels like it wakes up a little more and the act of writing helps me to put thoughts in order and work through my feelings. That has been much needed, especially as work has become stressful again.

It was that time of year again. Time for the annual project which had caused high levels of stress and disrupted my recovery last year. Despite the Event department receiving weekly updates on my progress, they decided to bring up their 'concerns over my work' in a meeting with the CEO.

'It is Friday, we needed those items from you this week.' Three expectant faces turned to me.

'The deadline you gave me for these items was the end of the year.' They nodded, still expectant. 'I'm on track to hand over these items in the last week of December.'

'No, the end of the year means the first week of December not the last.'

'What? In who's world is that true?'

With both of the Event team maintaining that their deadline wasn't confusing, there was nothing I could do without looking churlish. *Of course, no one would rely on the opinion of someone with a TBI.*

After the meeting, *ambush,* my department went to bat for me. Essentially there had been a mistake with the timeline and I made a handy fall guy. A few colleagues came up to say they agreed with my interpretation of an 'end of the year' deadline. But it was never said publicly and everyone was too busy to help. The Event manager had managed to pin the blame on someone outside her department. *Pick on the weak.* Perhaps she didn't stop to consider the doubt and damage that gaslighting someone on a graded return from brain injury would cause? Would she have foreseen the fear, the attributions? *Is this my fault? Will I always be the scapegoat now?*

These thoughts bounced around my head but I wasn't able to work through them as I was stuck in a project from hell. My three days of work bled at the edges. Food and cognitive breaks were missed, as I worked from dawn till dusk, fighting off dizziness and the grey fatigue that built inexorably. My alleged days off were spent logging in to the office servers from home. I managed snatches of work between hastily gulped down painkillers.

The meticulously detailed Fatigue Management Planner had gone out the window. Migraines grew and merged into a horrible contestant roar. Life outside the office stopped at the most social time of year. Finally, it was over and I sent the final documents with a weary sigh. The thanks I received for undermining my health again was 'At last, she delivers.' I found myself sitting alone at the office Christmas party feeling grey, stretched and thin. *I don't want to be here next year.*

Most of the bright spots that month were found in the snatched moments of rest. The migraines, fatigue and sheer volume of work meant that I missed many parties or catch-ups. However, I had been enjoying my time volunteering for the brain injury charity so was determined to make their Christmas party. I was exhausted so half-heatedly offered to help and ended up being the DJ. That was a bit of a poisoned chalice as the organisers wanted a big singalong, but a lot of background noise isn't the best thing in a brain injury meeting. In end it, it was a fun evening, with carols, food and bingo. I paid the price for my enthusiasm as I was very unwell for a few days. The world was spinning and I was nauseous and exhausted. *I've not felt this awful for a long time.* Too much work and not enough fun this year.

Diary entry

NEW YEAR'S EVE 2017: Despite putting the diary away earlier this year, I feel the need to mark the end of another year with another diary entry. Poetry has been a dalliance in my life rather than a constant love. I seem to have returned to it thanks to Judi Dench's rendition of Tennyson's Ulysses in the movie Skyfall which I watched yesterday.

> 'We are not now that strength which in old days
> Moved earth and heaven, that which we are, we are;
> One equal temper of heroic hearts,
> Made weak by time and fate, but strong in will
> To strive, to seek, to find, and not to yield.'

It is true that I am not now that strength which I used to be. I feel I am still coming to terms with the new reality of restrictions imposed on body and brain by the events of the last few years. I have been dwelling on my mortality a great deal. This is driven by the flashes of childhood memories which continue to return in my third year of recovery. They bring with them a deep yearning for what has passed. A homesickness made more melancholy in the knowledge that those happy times of childhood in the idyllic New Zealand countryside will never come again. Even were I to move back to that farmstead, so much has changed. Not least my perception of a wider world.

Recently, mum told us of their struggle through an economic crash in New Zealand. When she and dad just needed to get their heads down and get through it. None of that taints my memories. I was blissfully unaware as I charged around the paddocks and bush with my brother and sister. It is that which I miss most, that sense of happiness and innocence of the world as I know that can never come again.

When I said this to Ash, he reminded me that I'm not even half way through my expected life span. That news seemed wearisome at first, 'you mean there is more?!' But my turn to the Tennyson poem gives me the answer. I have not struggled through the helpless, hopeless and despairing times of the last few years only to dread the next few!

Yes, I have been 'made weak by time and fate.' But I am 'strong in will'. I will strive, and seek and find. And I will not yield.

References

Burgess, M. (2016). 'Rugby League: Lance Hohaia's nightmare head knocks. Originally published in the New Zealand Herald on Sunday on 20 March 2016 – written by NZME Sports Journalist Michael Burgess. Available at: https://www.nzherald.co.nz/sport/news/article.cfm?c_id=4&objectid=11608680

Tennyson, A. (1842). Poems, vol. 2. London: Moxon.

Chapter 17

Finding happiness within limitations

Who will I be?

2018

January: Three years and ten months after the incident

Summary of email from Hawthorn

ME: Happy New Year writing class. It is short notice but I have some exciting news and would like to meet you all on Thursday the fourth to discuss it.

Hawthorn had chosen the meeting spot carefully. One of the group still had mobility problems while we all struggled on busy public transport and with listening in loud environments. The generic chain cafe was on top of a tube station, fully accessible with lifts and had booths with high partitions to dull sounds.

We shared cheery greetings and ordered tea and scones. Our writing class had been meeting weekly for over a year now and every gathering involved snacks. It wasn't just my brain injury which functioned better with regular watering and feeding. After the first sips of tea had been savoured, conversation drew to a natural halt and we three students looked expectantly at the teacher.

'As you know, I was thrilled with the group story that we competed in the summer. I then wanted to see what it would look like as a play and we completed that in the autumn. Well, long story short, and through a few contacts, it came to the attention of a group putting on an exhibition at Tate Modern. The exhibit is in their interactive Tate Exchange gallery and they would like us to do a reading of our play in the gallery.'

Holy sh*t! The silence which greeted her announcement showed that I wasn't the only one stunned.

Hawthorn cleared her throat and continued. 'Umm, of course. It won't happen if you prefer it doesn't. This is a group exercise, so we need the whole group to agree.' More silence. 'Would someone like to say something? Please?'

Suddenly we all had questions.

'Our play? Are you sure?'

'At the Tate Modern?'

'When, what do we need to do?'

The animated meeting went on for an hour. We would be part of a week-long exploration of future communities taking place in a month's time. It was short notice, and we needed to find people prepared to read as our 'cast'. When the meeting broke up, we were happy, exhausted and determined to do it.

Quote from Hawthorn

> People have such an unfortunate reaction to brain injuries. This is a chance to show what everyone has to offer and to encourage understanding, awareness and kindness.

Email to parents

ME: Sorry I'm a bit manic at the moment, I'd only just started to recover from a frantic December when this Tate Modern opportunity came up. Plenty to organise as we are 'on' in two weeks. The good news is that I saw the neuro-otology clinic again. The dizzy docs said that, once I've recovered from these frantic weeks, I can start to reduce the trippy pills. Hurray! So sometime in April, I might be able to do evenings again!

February: Three years and eleven months after the incident

He cut an odd figure, hunched over and shuffling past the bus stop. The blue plastic sandals on his feet were a poor choice in the freezing weather. I was several metres away but could see that his lips were moving. *Is he asking that woman something?* The woman didn't break her stride and the man didn't seem to notice her pass by. *Guess not, ah well. Best not interfere, remember last time.*

Hours later I was walking to the bus stop again. *Huh, that man again.* The elderly gent was still walking past the bus stop, his blue sandals now covered in mud. *Odd, must be a glitch in the matrix.*

He turned and I saw his face. His cracked lips were still mumbling above a beard now caked in drool. Some of his whiskers were frozen stiff with it, elsewhere his saliva hung in long glistening strands. *Yeah best not interfere. How could I help anyway?*

Then I was close enough to see his face. *Oh no, those eyes.* The confusion and loss were bad enough. But beneath that I recognised a deep, paralysing fear. One that I had become far too familiar with in the early days after the incident. *Help him!* I stopped in his path; the sandals shuffled to a halt. Slowly, he focused on my face.

'Can I help you?'

His eyes flashed as he started to speak. *I was wrong, he's about to tell me to bugger off.* Then he paused. The fear was back and his lips trembled: 'Memory... bad.' Wrinkles on his craggy face dropped and he pointed urgently to his head. A hospital band fluttered around his wrist. 'Memory...' His mouth churned again, searching for the right word. 'Memory... bad.' He looked at me, more closely this time. Did I understand?

'Ok, well...' *Sh*t, what do I do?* '...umm, do you remember where you live?'

'Home, I was going home.' His eyes lit up, pleased to be able to recall that much. 'It's around here... somewhere.' His cracked lips started to bleed slightly. They had dried out from hours of walking in late winter cold and this conversation was taking its toll.

'Would you like a drink, I have some water?'

He nodded, but as I offered him the bottle, he ignored it and said. 'Home, I need to go home.' His voice was thin but carried. The pain in it gathered stares from those waiting for the bus nearby. Rush hour traffic blew dirt and old leaves into his face. Tears came back and his eyes scrunched up like a child's.

Not here, get him somewhere quiet. 'There is a park just around the corner where it is a little quieter and you can sit down.'

The threatened tears passed, he nodded eagerly and I took his hand. With the other I pulled my phone out and dialled the non-emergency police number.

Email to Maple

ME: I'm sorry I didn't make the catch up tonight, but really pleased I stopped to ask an old man if he was OK. I'd spotted him looking really haggard and drooling and he was still there five hours later, still pacing the same spot.

Turns out he was a dementia patient who had wandered out of hospital and forgotten the rest of the way home. When the ambulance turned up, he said 'wow' and shook my hand. It was a nice reminder that even our little gestures made a difference.

It had been a heck of a month and suddenly it was the night before our performance. I tried to relax but the brain was constantly whirring. Picking up a subject, worrying at it, thrashing through all the possible consequences of an action before throwing it away in frustration. I would tell myself to rest, to relax into the meditation of breathing and just being. It had worked before but it was so hard to do, when there was so much going on, when every moment you sat still half of you was thinking that there is more you must do.

My work will be at the Tate Modern tomorrow. I must prepare. I must be ready. I hadn't yet done my usual routine of worst-case-scenario thinking to work through all the possible outcomes and mini-crises that tomorrow promised. *How can I possibly relax when so much is left undone?* At times like this I could second guess myself and jump immediately to the worst possible outcome.

What if there is an explosion, do I know the best way out of the building? With everyone running for the stairs, could I climb down the outside from the fifth floor? I used this to show myself the ridiculous outcome of such thinking, to try and nip my anxious behaviour in the bud. But, through the mocking laughter in my head, part of me was thinking *Yes, reckon I could get out that way...*

Summary of newsletter from the local brain injury charity

A huge thank you to our teacher and to the amazing group of writers and their supporters who put together an inspirational presentation at the Tate Modern this weekend. The event was the public reading of a play which explores the effect of a brain injury on an individual and their loved ones. All writers in the group had suffered a brain injury and the work comes from their personal experiences. We hope our involvement with the event will communicate to those less familiar with brain injury and help them gain a better understanding of what happens to those who suffer such an injury.

March: Four years after the incident

Summary of emails with parents

ME: Morning from a thawed London. Never seen so much snow in the central city nor have it hang around for so long. You are right that the reason you haven't heard from me for a while is because I'm having a mini-collapse for my fourth anniversary. December was demanding at work, it would have been stressful for someone working full-time, let alone someone on a part-time graded return. It brought on migraines, dizziness and fatigue again, which I didn't really recover from over the Christmas break.

January & February were far busier than planned. The opportunity to put on the play was amazing, one of those 'once in a life time' things. I've done performance art at the Tate! It was a lot of work but I don't regret that for one second. It felt like exactly the kind of thing I want to be getting busy and excited about.

Work is a different matter. I'm putting the pressure on myself but also feeling disillusioned after the fiasco of the project deadline. And my insurance case has just dragged on with no answers for years now. It feels like I'm the only one interested in it sometimes. Certainly, it is clear that I'm caring more about work than work is about me. I seem to be spending all my energy on something I don't want to do, and it is interfering with things I do want to do. So am quietly contemplating if I could turn writing into my job…

MUM: Your reading was exciting, and we may have been bragging a little here, as all parents do. With the writing and the class continuing, perhaps it is time to do more than explore those thoughts?

When I was 38, I remember sitting in the garden and working out 'The Plan.' Where we, as a family, were headed and how to get there. Mortgage to be paid. Three to educate with tertiary education. Save for retirement. Holidays for us all. My wish for a good, well paid job and how I would retrain to find one. That was 'The Plan' and it worked.

Your sister landed her job with the civil service at 38, aced her training, and has flown up the ranks. Maybe 38 is the golden age for making the big decisions of taking the next step? For you to formulate a new career or life plan? So, I encourage you to seriously look at taking the next step. I am amazed at the number of folk who have taken a leap of faith and been delighted. Just wished they had done it sooner.

Remember Indiana Jones and the Holy Grail, when he had to step off the cliff and hope the path was there… and it was. It's all a bit like that. Lots of love xxxx

'I've been bragging too, I can't blame your parents at all. Can't believe I have photos of my friend doing performance art at the Tate.'

It was coffee and cake morning with Peony. This had become a monthly occasion on one of my days off. However, this was the first time since the reading that I'd been well enough to meet. It was a treat and I was going all out. The server arrived; his tray piled high with goodies.

'And whose is the "Red Velvet Chocolate Cake Coconut Milk Latte"?'

Peony dissolved. 'Wait, that's a thing?'

'You're damn right it's a thing, and now it is my thing.'

The ginormous cup settled in front of me, and the next few minutes were lost to photos, giggles and taste tests. Finally, Peony turned the conversation back to the writing class.

'So what is next for the play?'

'Well, the script is out with people, there's a writing festival in June… who knows?'

'That's amazing!'

I stared into my lake of coffee. *Tell her why you are worried.*

'You're worried about something.'

'Damn it, do I just wear my thoughts on my face now?'

'You always did, that's not new.'

'It's just… I want to do more, I want to tell people about brain injury and what it's like, and maybe, I dunno, it might help someone.'

'That's all good and noble-sounding, what's the problem?'

'It's just, I'm not sure I should. I mean, I'm not sure I'm the right person to. My injury was a mild TBI. That's the actual medical definition for it. Mild. I keep meeting people who are struggling to walk, or speak, or who have had to rebuild lives after months spent in comas or rehabilitation centres. I've never been admitted to hospital, had no obvious injuries apart from bruises and am back to b*tching about normal things. So how can I raise awareness of something I haven't had really badly?'

Peony put down her cup and leaned in. 'Listen up. What happened to you, what is still happening to you, is awful and traumatic. Don't belittle it by comparing yourself with others.'

'Thank you.'

She didn't move, watched me closely. *Damn, that was good to hear.* The relief must have shown on my face as she sat back and attacked her Pastéis de Nata. 'Good. Now that's sorted, what will you do?'

April: Four years and one month after the incident

Summary of emails with the company's new HR manager

ME: While I am interested in the proposed new role in the department, there are some issues which need to be resolved first. You may not be aware that the company are pursuing a case with their insurers over my injury in March 2014 and subsequent absence. My current contract was supposed to be temporary pending the outcome of the claim. The claim would hopefully lead to compensation to the company for sick-leave and other costs, and the re-instatement of my previous salary and benefits.

This claim was instigated three years ago, in the summer of 2015. I have been chasing the insurance representative for updates with little success over the years. I was told that your predecessor last spoke to the representative nearly eighteen months ago, at the end of 2016, and expressed displeasure at the lack of progress. However, we still have not had answers or requests for further information from the insurers. With the changes in HR, perhaps this can be resolved?

NEW HR MANAGER: I am sorry that it's taken more time than I would have preferred to respond in writing to you on this matter. As mentioned the other day, it's been difficult to achieve a conversation with the insurance representative, however, I am delighted to say that we have spoken today. I have been provided with a very brief overview which mirrors the details you have already given to me. The good news about that is that he's clued up to be able to have a meaningful conversation concerning your case.

We will be meeting in the middle of next month for a review on several matters, yours being part of the agenda. Between now and then he will attempt to make progress on the claim. He suspects that it may be placed back at the start position which will require an update with medical evidence, but don't hold me/us to that, I'm just sharing his opinion at present.

What? All these years, and now it's back to the start again? There was a flurry of activity from the insurance company that month, none of it prom-ising and most of it dismissive. The result can best be summed up as 'it was decided the case will not be pursued'.

'W*nkers!' Laurel fumed and stabbed at her salad. 'So, that's how they do it? Sit on the case for three years and then say "No, and it's too late to ask again."'

'So it would seem. It's disappointing, but glad I pushed for an answer. At least I have one now.'

'You are taking this rather well.'

'They're insurers, who part with money less readily than their teeth. What do you expect? The question for me is, what next?'

Laurel's eyes sparkled. 'And...? Are you going to do it?'

'It would mean I could actually recover properly and do what I want to do...'

'So, what are you waiting for?'

Letter to manager

> I would like to inform you that I am leaving my position with the company to pursue other interests. I will document recent changes for the next process of this project. In my eight years at the company I consider myself lucky to have worked alongside some excellent colleagues and to be involved in the company's immense growth.
>
> I also wish to express gratitude to you, the department team and to the wider corporation for the support, both formal and informal, offered following my brain injury and in the on-going recovery. Best wishes to you & everyone at the company and I do hope our paths will cross again in future.

Oh, crikey. What have I done?

May: Four years and two months after the incident

'So that is why you are looking so relaxed!'

I'd managed to meet Hazel for a rare catch up. She was busy with a new house and career so it had been a while since we had been able to meet.

'Yep, only seven days of work left now, but due to my part-time hours I'm not completely free for a few more weeks.'

'And what will you do instead?'

'I mean, it is a good question. I'm horrible to live with when bored, but the writing started to look very exciting.'

'Yes, the Tate thing sounded great. I'm sorry I couldn't see your play.'

'You might get a chance yet, the writing group is invited to a summer festival. It's exciting but we need to triple the length of the play before then!'

'So that still has wheels. What about the dosh problem?'

'Well, we should be ok, despite the insurance not coming through. To help that along I'm getting in touch with local charities to see what they do and if they need content writers. My writing teacher is also keen to see something happen with my fiction stories.'

'So, competitions and things?'

'Uh huh. Of course, it will take a while for this to start building the bank balance. Fortunately, Ash has recently become a permanent staff member rather than on contract, so things are a bit more secure right now.'

'That's the key thing.'

'Yes, without that, this would have been much harder. As it is, I'm pleased I've quit work as don't know how I'd have fit it all in!'

'And all because of the brain injury. Will you write about that?'

Reference

Hawthorne, C. (2018). *Personal communication*, 4 January 2018.

Epilogue
Me, but different

8th July 2018: Four years and four months after the incident

'Aaaand Go!'

I jump onto the first stump and leap to the next, then a third. *I can do this. Only a few more stumps to the rope bridge, and then on to the balance beam.*

It is early morning and we have come to the park with Maple's toddler. He is playing happily in the sand pit, this amazing new person who will never know me without a brain injury. Rose is over from the United States for a visit and the three of us are running off the cobwebs of a late night. It has been many years since we first met, and time has changed us all. But we are still competitive and a timed race round the playground obstacles was inevitable.

Rose ran first and set a fast pace, as a natural runner she is usually in the lead. I am determined to catch her. Sun sparkles off the late dew but I ignore the glint and make a strong start on the rope bridge. The planks groan under my thudding steps, they aren't used to an adult running across them. The bridge sags as I reach the middle and the gentle shivers turn to a wild sway. I feel a familiar but faint echo of motion in my ear and wobble, my pace slows down. Rose and Maple give a chorus of encouragement.

'Halfway-split, you are just behind!'

'C'mon, you can win this!'

I reach the end of the bridge and enjoy the solidity of the balance beam after the moving bridge. After the first few steps, the dizziness in my ear fades and I pick up speed again. *A few more steps and...*

'Time!' we all shout as my feet hit the finish line.

'So close!'

'Aww, man. You were only five seconds off the pace.'

'Noooooo!' I sink to the ground in defeat. 'Robbed, I was robbed.'

'Ok, now time me.' Maple is keen to challenge for the title. I stand to take the timer and a wave of dizziness rolls through my head. It is gone quickly but leaves me lightheaded and weak. I sink on to the park bench to recover.

'You ok?'

'Yeah, fine.' I smile up at my friends. 'Just need a moment.'

Rose passes me a water bottle. Maple looks me up and down then: 'You know, I forget there's anything wrong. Now and then I have to remind myself that you had a brain injury and need to stop occasionally.'

Only someone who had known me for a long time would see past the changes and know that I was back to just me. Me, but different. The recovery isn't over, I will always carry those scars in my head. But life isn't over either. It is time to get out there, scars and all.

References

Burgess, M. (2016). *'Rugby League: Lance Hohaia's Nightmare Head Knocks.* Originally published in the New Zealand Herald on Sunday on 20 March 2016 – written by NZME Sports Journalist Michael Burgess. Available at: https://www. nzherald.co.nz/sport/news/article.cfm?c_id=4&objectid=11608680

Carroll, L. (1865). *Alice's Adventures in Wonderland*. London: Macmillan

Hawking, S. (2016). *The Reith Lectures. Professor Stephen Hawking: Black Holes, Episode 2 'Black Holes Ain't as Black As they Are Painted.'* BBC Radio 4, first transmitted 2 February 2016. Available at: https://www.bbc.co.uk/programmes/ b06qjzv8

Hawthorne, C. (2018). Personal communication.

Headway – The Brain Injury Association (2014). *Rehabilitation after Brain Injury*. www.headway.org.uk. Available at: https://www.headway.org.uk/about-brain-injury/individuals/rehabilitation-and-continuing-care/rehabilitation/ Last accessed May 2020.

Seemungal, B. (2017). *Imbalance and Dizziness after Brain Injury*.

Tennyson, A. (1842). *Poems, Vol. 2*. London: Moxon.

Glossary

NB: these are not medical definitions, rather they are simplified explanations from a layperson's perspective.

ABI see *Acquired Brain Injury*

Acquired Brain Injury An injury caused to the brain after birth which may be caused by external forces like a fall or an accident or by something internal, like a tumour or stroke.

Amitriptyline A medicine which was prescribed to the author in order to prevent migraines, also known as a *migraine prophylactic*. Amitriptyline is also used to treat pain and depression and can come in tablet or liquid form. Sometimes referred to in this book as *trippy pills*.

Anonymous FC The opposition football team during the game in which the author was injured.

Brain injury survivor A person living with the effects of an injury to their brain.

Cavernous haemangioma A small tangle of weakened blood vessels in the brain.

City United The football team the author was playing for when she was injured.

CBT *see Cognitive behavioral therapy*

Cognitive behavioural therapy A therapy which involves changing habits of behaviour and thinking. It is used to treat depression, anxiety disorders and some medical conditions.

Cognitive lapse A lapse in memory or concentration, sometimes called memory lapse or a 'senior moment'.

Concussion An injury to the brain caused by a blow to the head or sudden shaking of the neck and head. Usually lasts only a few days or weeks but can last longer and become *post-concussion syndrome*. This is also a *mild traumatic brain injury* and an *acquired brain injury*.

Contrast MRI   A *magnetic resonance imaging (MRI)* scan where a contrasting dye is injected into the body to highlight blood vessels or certain tissues on the resulting images.

Dizzy doctors   see *Neuro-otology*.

False attributions   When a person with a brain injury assumes that the difficulty they are experiencing is due solely to their injury.

Fatigue Management planner   A calendar upon which a person experiencing cognitive fatigue can plan their daily and weekly tasks in order to balance activities with rest.

Four P's of Fatigue Management   Perspective, Priorities, Planning and Pacing.

General Practitioner or GP   The patient's local doctor.

IAM   see *Internal auditory meatus*.

The incident   The day on which the author's injury occurred, 9 March 2014.

Internal auditory meatus   A canal through part of the skull near the inner ear. Also known as the meatus acusticus internus, internal acoustic meatus, internal auditory canal, or internal acoustic canal.

Magnetic resonance imaging (MRI)   A medical scan which uses strong magnetic fields and radio waves to produce detailed images of the inside of the body.

Migraine diary   A record of when and where migraines hit including what you were doing at the time and just before the migraine. This can help to identify the triggers and monitor how well any medicine or other preventative steps are working.

Migraine prophylactic   A medicine which can help to prevent migraines. The author was prescribed *amitriptyline*, though other medications are used.

Mild TBI   see *Mild traumatic brain injury*

Mild traumatic brain injury   A *traumatic brain injury* is considered 'mild' in severity when there is no loss of consciousness, or if the person is unconscious for less than half an hour. If any *post-traumatic amnesia* occurs, then a brain injury is considered mild if the disorientation does not continue beyond 24 hours.

Minor head injury   see *Concussion*.

Neuro-otology   The diagnosis, investigation, management and rehabilitation of disorders associated with the *vestibular system*. Sometimes referred to in the narrative as *dizzy doctors*.

Neuropsychology   The study of how brain function affects behaviour, emotion, and cognition, and vice versa.

Neuro-rehabilitation   A series of therapies which aim to improve brain function and improve the wellbeing of people with diseases, trauma or disorders of the nervous system, including people with brain injuries.

Post-traumatic amnesia   The period of time after an injury when a person is conscious but is behaving or talking in strange manner.

River FC   The football club which the author worked with during her recovery where she helped to create a women's team.

TBI   see *traumatic brain injury.*

Traumatic brain injury   An injury to the brain caused by a head injury, is also an *acquired brain injury.*

Tinnitus   The sensation of hearing a noise even when the environment is silent. The noise, usually a buzz or a ringing sound, is generated by a person's own auditory system.

Vestibular migraines   A type of severe headache which occurs more than once in which the person feels dizzy as well as severe pain. The attacks can last anywhere for as short as three hours to as long as three days. Is also known as migrainous vertigo or migraine associated dizziness.

Vestibular physiotherapy   A series of exercises designed to reduce dizziness and improve a person's balance.

Vocational rehabilitation   A service to assist a person with chronic disease or who is recovering from a disease or injury to remain in, or return to, employment safely.

Index

For Product Safety Concerns and Information please contact our EU
representative GPSR@taylorandfrancis.com
Taylor & Francis Verlag GmbH, Kaufingerstraße 24, 80331 München, Germany

www.ingramcontent.com/pod-product-compliance
Ingram Content Group UK Ltd.
Pitfield, Milton Keynes, MK11 3LW, UK
UKHW021425080625
459435UK00011B/162